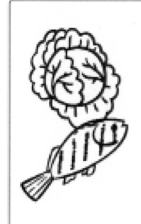
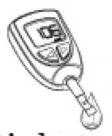
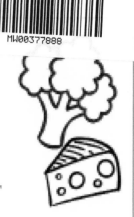

# This Diabetes & Food Journal Belongs To:

- - - - - - - - - - - - - - - - - - - - - - - - - - - - - - - - - - - - - - -

This journal is designed to help you manage your diet controlled diabetes.

Keeping a food journal along with your daily readings helps you to learn which foods are causing you issues with glucose levels going too high. You'll learn that certain foods need to be avoided and which ones you can have in moderation.

Controlling one's diabetes is a lifelong journey and not always easy. This journal can help you manage your diabetes to keep your A1C Levels down and to live a healthier life.

# Foods To Avoid
Use this page to list foods that cause glucose spikes

# Foods To Avoid
Use this page to list foods that cause glucose spikes

_____

_____

_____

_____

_____

_____

_____

_____

_____

_____

_____

_____

_____

_____

_____

_____

Date:_____

A.M. Glucose Reading:_____

---

Breakfast:

Time:_____ Total Carbs:_____

_____

_____

Two Hour Glucose Reading:_____
Mid Morning Snack:_____

---

Lunch:

Time:_____ Total Carbs:_____

_____

_____

Two Hour Glucose Reading:_____
Mid Afternoon Snack:_____

---

Dinner:

Time:_____Total Carbs:_____

_____

_____

Two Hour Glucose Reading:_____
Evening Snack:_____

Date:_____

A.M. Glucose Reading:_____

Breakfast:

Time:_____    Total Carbs:_____

_____

_____

_____

Two Hour Glucose Reading:_____

Mid Morning Snack:_____

Lunch:

Time:_____    Total Carbs:_____

_____

_____

_____

Two Hour Glucose Reading:_____

Mid Afternoon Snack:_____

Dinner:

Time:_____    Total Carbs:_____

_____

_____

_____

Two Hour Glucose Reading:_____

Evening Snack:_____

Date:_____

A.M. Glucose Reading:_____

Breakfast:

Time:_____ Total Carbs:_____

_____
_____
_____

Two Hour Glucose Reading:_____
Mid Morning Snack:_____

Lunch:

Time:_____ Total Carbs:_____

_____
_____
_____

Two Hour Glucose Reading:_____
Mid Afternoon Snack:_____

Dinner:

Time:_____Total Carbs:_____

_____
_____
_____

Two Hour Glucose Reading:_____
Evening Snack:_____

Date:_____

A.M. Glucose Reading:_____

Breakfast:

Time:_____   Total Carbs:_____

_____

_____

_____

Two Hour Glucose Reading:_____

Mid Morning Snack:_____

Lunch:

Time:_____   Total Carbs:_____

_____

_____

_____

Two Hour Glucose Reading:_____

Mid Afternoon Snack:_____

Dinner:

Time:_____Total Carbs:_____

_____

_____

_____

Two Hour Glucose Reading:_____

Evening Snack:_____

Date:_____

A.M. Glucose Reading:_____

---

Breakfast:

Time:_____    Total Carbs:_____

_____
_____
_____

Two Hour Glucose Reading:_____
Mid Morning Snack:_____

---

Lunch:

Time:_____    Total Carbs:_____

_____
_____
_____

Two Hour Glucose Reading:_____
Mid Afternoon Snack:_____

---

Dinner:

Time:_____Total Carbs:_____

_____
_____
_____

Two Hour Glucose Reading:_____
Evening Snack:_____

Date:_____

A.M. Glucose Reading:_____

Breakfast:

Time:_____ Total Carbs:_____

_____

_____

_____

Two Hour Glucose Reading:_____

Mid Morning Snack:_____

Lunch:

Time:_____ Total Carbs:_____

_____

_____

_____

Two Hour Glucose Reading:_____

Mid Afternoon Snack:_____

Dinner:

Time:_____Total Carbs:_____

_____

_____

_____

Two Hour Glucose Reading:_____

Evening Snack:_____

Date:_____

A.M. Glucose Reading:_____

---

Breakfast:

Time:_____ Total Carbs:_____

_____
_____
_____

Two Hour Glucose Reading:_____
Mid Morning Snack:_____

---

Lunch:

Time:_____ Total Carbs:_____

_____
_____
_____

Two Hour Glucose Reading:_____
Mid Afternoon Snack:_____

---

Dinner:

Time:_____Total Carbs:_____

_____
_____
_____

Two Hour Glucose Reading:_____
Evening Snack:_____

Date:_____

A.M. Glucose Reading:_____

Breakfast:

Time:_____ Total Carbs:_____
_____
_____
_____

Two Hour Glucose Reading:_____
Mid Morning Snack:_____

Lunch:

Time:_____ Total Carbs:_____
_____
_____
_____

Two Hour Glucose Reading:_____
Mid Afternoon Snack:_____

Dinner:

Time:_____Total Carbs:_____
_____
_____
_____

Two Hour Glucose Reading:_____
Evening Snack:_____

Date:_____

A.M. Glucose Reading:_____

Breakfast:

Time:_____ Total Carbs:_____

_____
_____
_____

Two Hour Glucose Reading:_____
Mid Morning Snack:_____

Lunch:

Time:_____ Total Carbs:_____

_____
_____
_____

Two Hour Glucose Reading:_____
Mid Afternoon Snack:_____

Dinner:

Time:_____Total Carbs:_____

_____
_____
_____

Two Hour Glucose Reading:_____
Evening Snack:_____

Date:_____

A.M. Glucose Reading:_____

Breakfast:

Time:_____ Total Carbs:_____

_____

_____

_____

Two Hour Glucose Reading:_____

Mid Morning Snack:_____

Lunch:

Time:_____ Total Carbs:_____

_____

_____

_____

Two Hour Glucose Reading:_____

Mid Afternoon Snack:_____

Dinner:

Time:_____Total Carbs:_____

_____

_____

_____

Two Hour Glucose Reading:_____

Evening Snack:_____

Date:_____

A.M. Glucose Reading:_____

---

Breakfast:

Time:_____ Total Carbs:_____

_____

_____

_____

Two Hour Glucose Reading:_____

Mid Morning Snack:_____

---

Lunch:

Time:_____ Total Carbs:_____

_____

_____

_____

Two Hour Glucose Reading:_____

Mid Afternoon Snack:_____

---

Dinner:

Time:_____Total Carbs:_____

_____

_____

_____

Two Hour Glucose Reading:_____

Evening Snack:_____

Date:_____

A.M. Glucose Reading:_____

Breakfast:

Time:_____ Total Carbs:_____

_____
_____
_____

Two Hour Glucose Reading:_____
Mid Morning Snack:_____

Lunch:

Time:_____ Total Carbs:_____

_____
_____
_____

Two Hour Glucose Reading:_____
Mid Afternoon Snack:_____

Dinner:

Time:_____Total Carbs:_____

_____
_____
_____

Two Hour Glucose Reading:_____
Evening Snack:_____

Date:_____

A.M. Glucose Reading:_____

Breakfast:

Time:_____ Total Carbs:_____

_____

_____

_____

Two Hour Glucose Reading:_____

Mid Morning Snack:_____

Lunch:

Time:_____ Total Carbs:_____

_____

_____

_____

Two Hour Glucose Reading:_____

Mid Afternoon Snack:_____

Dinner:

Time:_____Total Carbs:_____

_____

_____

_____

Two Hour Glucose Reading:_____

Evening Snack:_____

Date:_____

A.M. Glucose Reading:_____

Breakfast:

Time:_____ Total Carbs:_____

_____

_____

_____

Two Hour Glucose Reading:_____

Mid Morning Snack:_____

Lunch:

Time:_____ Total Carbs:_____

_____

_____

_____

Two Hour Glucose Reading:_____

Mid Afternoon Snack:_____

Dinner:

Time:_____Total Carbs:_____

_____

_____

_____

Two Hour Glucose Reading:_____

Evening Snack:_____

Date:_____

A.M. Glucose Reading:_____

Breakfast:

Time:_____ Total Carbs:_____

_____
_____
_____

Two Hour Glucose Reading:_____
Mid Morning Snack:_____

Lunch:

Time:_____ Total Carbs:_____

_____
_____
_____

Two Hour Glucose Reading:_____
Mid Afternoon Snack:_____

Dinner:

Time:_____ Total Carbs:_____

_____
_____
_____

Two Hour Glucose Reading:_____
Evening Snack:_____

Date:_____

A.M. Glucose Reading:_____

Breakfast:

Time:_____  Total Carbs:_____

_____

_____

_____

Two Hour Glucose Reading:_____

Mid Morning Snack:_____

Lunch:

Time:_____  Total Carbs:_____

_____

_____

_____

Two Hour Glucose Reading:_____
Mid Afternoon Snack:_____

Dinner:

Time:_____Total Carbs:_____

_____

_____

_____

Two Hour Glucose Reading:_____
Evening Snack:_____

Date:_____

A.M. Glucose Reading:_____

Breakfast:

Time:_____   Total Carbs:_____

_____
_____
_____

Two Hour Glucose Reading:_____
Mid Morning Snack:_____

Lunch:

Time:_____   Total Carbs:_____

_____
_____
_____

Two Hour Glucose Reading:_____
Mid Afternoon Snack:_____

Dinner:

Time:_____Total Carbs:_____

_____
_____
_____

Two Hour Glucose Reading:_____
Evening Snack:_____

Date:_____

A.M. Glucose Reading:_____

Breakfast:

Time:_____ Total Carbs:_____

_____
_____
_____

Two Hour Glucose Reading:_____
Mid Morning Snack:_____

Lunch:

Time:_____ Total Carbs:_____

_____
_____
_____

Two Hour Glucose Reading:_____
Mid Afternoon Snack:_____

Dinner:

Time:_____Total Carbs:_____

_____
_____
_____

Two Hour Glucose Reading:_____
Evening Snack:_____

Date:_____

A.M. Glucose Reading:_____

Breakfast:

Time:_____ Total Carbs:_____

_____

_____

_____

Two Hour Glucose Reading:_____

Mid Morning Snack:_____

Lunch:

Time:_____ Total Carbs:_____

_____

_____

_____

Two Hour Glucose Reading:_____

Mid Afternoon Snack:_____

Dinner:

Time:_____Total Carbs:_____

_____

_____

_____

Two Hour Glucose Reading:_____

Evening Snack:_____

Date:_____

A.M. Glucose Reading:_____

Breakfast:

Time:_____ Total Carbs:_____

_____

_____

_____

Two Hour Glucose Reading:_____

Mid Morning Snack:_____

Lunch:

Time:_____ Total Carbs:_____

_____

_____

_____

Two Hour Glucose Reading:_____

Mid Afternoon Snack:_____

Dinner:

Time:_____ Total Carbs:_____

_____

_____

_____

Two Hour Glucose Reading:_____

Evening Snack:_____

Date:_____

A.M. Glucose Reading:_____

Breakfast:

Time:_____  Total Carbs:_____

_____

_____

_____

Two Hour Glucose Reading:_____

Mid Morning Snack:_____

Lunch:

Time:_____  Total Carbs:_____

_____

_____

_____

Two Hour Glucose Reading:_____
Mid Afternoon Snack:_____

Dinner:

Time:_____Total Carbs:_____

_____

_____

_____

Two Hour Glucose Reading:_____
Evening Snack:_____

Date:_____

A.M. Glucose Reading:_____

Breakfast:

Time:_____    Total Carbs:_____

_____
_____
_____

Two Hour Glucose Reading:_____
Mid Morning Snack:_____

Lunch:

Time:_____    Total Carbs:_____

_____
_____
_____

Two Hour Glucose Reading:_____
Mid Afternoon Snack:_____

Dinner:

Time:_____  Total Carbs:_____

_____
_____
_____

Two Hour Glucose Reading:_____
Evening Snack:_____

Date:_____

A.M. Glucose Reading:_____

---

Breakfast:

Time:_____  Total Carbs:_____

_____

_____

_____

Two Hour Glucose Reading:_____

Mid Morning Snack:_____

---

Lunch:

Time:_____  Total Carbs:_____

_____

_____

_____

Two Hour Glucose Reading:_____

Mid Afternoon Snack:_____

---

Dinner:

Time:_____Total Carbs:_____

_____

_____

_____

Two Hour Glucose Reading:_____

Evening Snack:_____

Date:_____

A.M. Glucose Reading:_____

Breakfast:

Time:_____ Total Carbs:_____

_____
_____
_____

Two Hour Glucose Reading:_____
Mid Morning Snack:_____

Lunch:

Time:_____ Total Carbs:_____

_____
_____
_____

Two Hour Glucose Reading:_____
Mid Afternoon Snack:_____

Dinner:

Time:_____ Total Carbs:_____

_____
_____
_____

Two Hour Glucose Reading:_____
Evening Snack:_____

Date:_____

A.M. Glucose Reading:_____

Breakfast:

Time:_____ Total Carbs:_____
_____
_____
_____
Two Hour Glucose Reading:_____
Mid Morning Snack:_____

Lunch:

Time:_____ Total Carbs:_____
_____
_____
_____
Two Hour Glucose Reading:_____
Mid Afternoon Snack:_____

Dinner:

Time:_____Total Carbs:_____
_____
_____
_____
Two Hour Glucose Reading:_____
Evening Snack:_____

Date:_____

A.M. Glucose Reading:_____

Breakfast:

Time:_____ Total Carbs:_____
_____
_____
_____

Two Hour Glucose Reading:_____
Mid Morning Snack:_____

Lunch:

Time:_____ Total Carbs:_____
_____
_____
_____

Two Hour Glucose Reading:_____
Mid Afternoon Snack:_____

Dinner:

Time:_____Total Carbs:_____
_____
_____
_____

Two Hour Glucose Reading:_____
Evening Snack:_____

Date:_____

A.M. Glucose Reading:_____

Breakfast:

Time:_____ Total Carbs:_____
_____
_____
_____

Two Hour Glucose Reading:_____
Mid Morning Snack:_____

Lunch:

Time:_____ Total Carbs:_____
_____
_____
_____

Two Hour Glucose Reading:_____
Mid Afternoon Snack:_____

Dinner:

Time:_____Total Carbs:_____
_____
_____
_____

Two Hour Glucose Reading:_____
Evening Snack:_____

Date:_____

A.M. Glucose Reading:_____

Breakfast:

Time:_____ Total Carbs:_____

_____

_____

_____

Two Hour Glucose Reading:_____

Mid Morning Snack:_____

Lunch:

Time:_____ Total Carbs:_____

_____

_____

_____

Two Hour Glucose Reading:_____

Mid Afternoon Snack:_____

Dinner:

Time:_____Total Carbs:_____

_____

_____

_____

Two Hour Glucose Reading:_____

Evening Snack:_____

Date:_____

A.M. Glucose Reading:_____

Breakfast:

Time:_____    Total Carbs:_____

_____
_____
_____

Two Hour Glucose Reading:_____
Mid Morning Snack:_____

Lunch:

Time:_____    Total Carbs:_____

_____
_____
_____

Two Hour Glucose Reading:_____
Mid Afternoon Snack:_____

Dinner:

Time:_____    Total Carbs:_____

_____
_____
_____

Two Hour Glucose Reading:_____
Evening Snack:_____

Date:_____

A.M. Glucose Reading:_____

Breakfast:

Time:_____ Total Carbs:_____

_____

_____

_____

Two Hour Glucose Reading:_____

Mid Morning Snack:_____

Lunch:

Time:_____ Total Carbs:_____

_____

_____

_____

Two Hour Glucose Reading:_____

Mid Afternoon Snack:_____

Dinner:

Time:_____Total Carbs:_____

_____

_____

_____

Two Hour Glucose Reading:_____

Evening Snack:_____

Date:_____

A.M. Glucose Reading:_____

Breakfast:

Time:_____ Total Carbs:_____

_____

_____

_____

Two Hour Glucose Reading:_____

Mid Morning Snack:_____

Lunch:

Time:_____ Total Carbs:_____

_____

_____

_____

Two Hour Glucose Reading:_____

Mid Afternoon Snack:_____

Dinner:

Time:_____Total Carbs:_____

_____

_____

_____

Two Hour Glucose Reading:_____

Evening Snack:_____

Date:_____

A.M. Glucose Reading:_____

Breakfast:

Time:_____ Total Carbs:_____
_____
_____
_____

Two Hour Glucose Reading:_____
Mid Morning Snack:_____

Lunch:

Time:_____ Total Carbs:_____
_____
_____
_____

Two Hour Glucose Reading:_____
Mid Afternoon Snack:_____

Dinner:

Time:_____Total Carbs:_____
_____
_____
_____

Two Hour Glucose Reading:_____
Evening Snack:_____

Date:_____

 A.M. Glucose Reading:_____

Breakfast:

Time:_____ Total Carbs:_____

_____
_____
_____

Two Hour Glucose Reading:_____
Mid Morning Snack:_____

Lunch:

Time:_____ Total Carbs:_____

_____
_____
_____

Two Hour Glucose Reading:_____
Mid Afternoon Snack:_____

Dinner:

Time:_____Total Carbs:_____

_____
_____
_____

Two Hour Glucose Reading:_____
Evening Snack:_____

Date:_____

A.M. Glucose Reading:_____

Breakfast:

Time:_____  Total Carbs:_____

_____

_____

_____

Two Hour Glucose Reading:_____

Mid Morning Snack:_____

Lunch:

Time:_____  Total Carbs:_____

_____

_____

_____

Two Hour Glucose Reading:_____

Mid Afternoon Snack:_____

Dinner:

Time:_____Total Carbs:_____

_____

_____

_____

Two Hour Glucose Reading:_____

Evening Snack:_____

Date:_____

A.M. Glucose Reading:_____

Breakfast:

Time:_____    Total Carbs:_____
_____
_____
_____

Two Hour Glucose Reading:_____
Mid Morning Snack:_____

Lunch:

Time:_____    Total Carbs:_____
_____
_____
_____

Two Hour Glucose Reading:_____
Mid Afternoon Snack:_____

Dinner:

Time:_____    Total Carbs:_____
_____
_____
_____

Two Hour Glucose Reading:_____
Evening Snack:_____

Date:_____

A.M. Glucose Reading:_____

Breakfast:

Time:_____ Total Carbs:_____

_____

_____

_____

Two Hour Glucose Reading:_____

Mid Morning Snack:_____

Lunch:

Time:_____ Total Carbs:_____

_____

_____

_____

Two Hour Glucose Reading:_____

Mid Afternoon Snack:_____

Dinner:

Time:_____Total Carbs:_____

_____

_____

_____

Two Hour Glucose Reading:_____

Evening Snack:_____

Date:_____

A.M. Glucose Reading:_____

Breakfast:

Time:_____ Total Carbs:_____

_____
_____
_____

Two Hour Glucose Reading:_____
Mid Morning Snack:_____

Lunch:

Time:_____ Total Carbs:_____

_____
_____
_____

Two Hour Glucose Reading:_____
Mid Afternoon Snack:_____

Dinner:

Time:_____Total Carbs:_____

_____
_____
_____

Two Hour Glucose Reading:_____
Evening Snack:_____

Date:_____

A.M. Glucose Reading:_____

Breakfast:

Time:_____ Total Carbs:_____
_____
_____
_____

Two Hour Glucose Reading:_____
Mid Morning Snack:_____

Lunch:

Time:_____ Total Carbs:_____
_____
_____
_____

Two Hour Glucose Reading:_____
Mid Afternoon Snack:_____

Dinner:

Time:_____Total Carbs:_____
_____
_____
_____

Two Hour Glucose Reading:_____
Evening Snack:_____

Date:_____

A.M. Glucose Reading:_____

Breakfast:

Time:_____  Total Carbs:_____

_____
_____
_____

Two Hour Glucose Reading:_____

Mid Morning Snack:_____

Lunch:

Time:_____  Total Carbs:_____

_____
_____
_____

Two Hour Glucose Reading:_____

Mid Afternoon Snack:_____

Dinner:

Time:_____Total Carbs:_____

_____
_____
_____

Two Hour Glucose Reading:_____

Evening Snack:_____

Date:_____

A.M. Glucose Reading:_____

---

Breakfast:

Time:_____ Total Carbs:_____

_____
_____
_____

Two Hour Glucose Reading:_____
Mid Morning Snack:_____

---

Lunch:

Time:_____ Total Carbs:_____

_____
_____
_____

Two Hour Glucose Reading:_____
Mid Afternoon Snack:_____

---

Dinner:

Time:_____Total Carbs:_____

_____
_____
_____

Two Hour Glucose Reading:_____
Evening Snack:_____

Date:_____

A.M. Glucose Reading:_____

Breakfast:

Time:_____ Total Carbs:_____

_____

_____

_____

Two Hour Glucose Reading:_____

Mid Morning Snack:_____

Lunch:

Time:_____ Total Carbs:_____

_____

_____

_____

Two Hour Glucose Reading:_____

Mid Afternoon Snack:_____

Dinner:

Time:_____ Total Carbs:_____

_____

_____

_____

Two Hour Glucose Reading:_____

Evening Snack:_____

Date:_____

A.M. Glucose Reading:_____

Breakfast:

Time:_____ Total Carbs:_____

_____

_____

_____

Two Hour Glucose Reading:_____

Mid Morning Snack:_____

Lunch:

Time:_____ Total Carbs:_____

_____

_____

_____

Two Hour Glucose Reading:_____

Mid Afternoon Snack:_____

Dinner:

Time:_____Total Carbs:_____

_____

_____

_____

Two Hour Glucose Reading:_____

Evening Snack:_____

Date:_____

A.M. Glucose Reading:_____

Breakfast:

Time:_____ Total Carbs:_____

_____
_____
_____

Two Hour Glucose Reading:_____
Mid Morning Snack:_____

Lunch:

Time:_____ Total Carbs:_____

_____
_____
_____

Two Hour Glucose Reading:_____
Mid Afternoon Snack:_____

Dinner:

Time:_____Total Carbs:_____

_____
_____
_____

Two Hour Glucose Reading:_____
Evening Snack:_____

Date:_____

A.M. Glucose Reading:_____

Breakfast:

Time:_____ Total Carbs:_____

_____

_____

_____

Two Hour Glucose Reading:_____

Mid Morning Snack:_____

Lunch:

Time:_____ Total Carbs:_____

_____

_____

_____

Two Hour Glucose Reading:_____

Mid Afternoon Snack:_____

Dinner:

Time:_____Total Carbs:_____

_____

_____

_____

Two Hour Glucose Reading:_____

Evening Snack:_____

Date:_____

A.M. Glucose Reading:_____

Breakfast:

Time:_____    Total Carbs:_____

_____
_____
_____

Two Hour Glucose Reading:_____
Mid Morning Snack:_____

Lunch:

Time:_____    Total Carbs:_____

_____
_____
_____

Two Hour Glucose Reading:_____
Mid Afternoon Snack:_____

Dinner:

Time:_____Total Carbs:_____

_____
_____
_____

Two Hour Glucose Reading:_____
Evening Snack:_____

Date:_____

A.M. Glucose Reading:_____

Breakfast:

Time:_____ Total Carbs:_____
_____
_____
_____

Two Hour Glucose Reading:_____

Mid Morning Snack:_____

Lunch:

Time:_____ Total Carbs:_____
_____
_____
_____

Two Hour Glucose Reading:_____

Mid Afternoon Snack:_____

Dinner:

Time:_____Total Carbs:_____
_____
_____
_____

Two Hour Glucose Reading:_____

Evening Snack:_____

Date:_____

A.M. Glucose Reading:_____

Breakfast:

Time:_____ Total Carbs:_____

_____

_____

_____

Two Hour Glucose Reading:_____

Mid Morning Snack:_____

Lunch:

Time:_____ Total Carbs:_____

_____

_____

_____

Two Hour Glucose Reading:_____
Mid Afternoon Snack:_____

Dinner:

Time:_____Total Carbs:_____

_____

_____

_____

Two Hour Glucose Reading:_____
Evening Snack:_____

Date:_____

A.M. Glucose Reading:_____

---

Breakfast:

Time:_____ Total Carbs:_____

_____
_____
_____

Two Hour Glucose Reading:_____

Mid Morning Snack:_____

---

Lunch:

Time:_____ Total Carbs:_____

_____
_____
_____

Two Hour Glucose Reading:_____

Mid Afternoon Snack:_____

---

Dinner:

Time:_____Total Carbs:_____

_____
_____
_____

Two Hour Glucose Reading:_____

Evening Snack:_____

Date:_____

A.M. Glucose Reading:_____

Breakfast:

Time:_____ Total Carbs:_____

_____
_____
_____

Two Hour Glucose Reading:_____

Mid Morning Snack:_____

Lunch:

Time:_____ Total Carbs:_____

_____
_____
_____

Two Hour Glucose Reading:_____
Mid Afternoon Snack:_____

Dinner:

Time:_____Total Carbs:_____

_____
_____
_____

Two Hour Glucose Reading:_____
Evening Snack:_____

Date:_____

A.M. Glucose Reading:_____

---

Breakfast:

Time:_____  Total Carbs:_____

_____
_____
_____

Two Hour Glucose Reading:_____
Mid Morning Snack:_____

---

Lunch:

Time:_____  Total Carbs:_____

_____
_____
_____

Two Hour Glucose Reading:_____
Mid Afternoon Snack:_____

---

Dinner:

Time:_____Total Carbs:_____

_____
_____
_____

Two Hour Glucose Reading:_____
Evening Snack:_____

Date:_____

A.M. Glucose Reading:_____

Breakfast:

Time:_____  Total Carbs:_____

_____

_____

_____

Two Hour Glucose Reading:_____

Mid Morning Snack:_____

Lunch:

Time:_____  Total Carbs:_____

_____

_____

_____

Two Hour Glucose Reading:_____

Mid Afternoon Snack:_____

Dinner:

Time:_____Total Carbs:_____

_____

_____

_____

Two Hour Glucose Reading:_____

Evening Snack:_____

Date:_____

A.M. Glucose Reading:_____

Breakfast:

Time:_____ Total Carbs:_____

_____

_____

_____

Two Hour Glucose Reading:_____

Mid Morning Snack:_____

Lunch:

Time:_____ Total Carbs:_____

_____

_____

_____

Two Hour Glucose Reading:_____

Mid Afternoon Snack:_____

Dinner:

Time:_____Total Carbs:_____

_____

_____

_____

Two Hour Glucose Reading:_____

Evening Snack:_____

Date:_____

A.M. Glucose Reading:_____

Breakfast:

Time:_____  Total Carbs:_____

_____

_____

_____

Two Hour Glucose Reading:_____

Mid Morning Snack:_____

Lunch:

Time:_____  Total Carbs:_____

_____

_____

_____

Two Hour Glucose Reading:_____

Mid Afternoon Snack:_____

Dinner:

Time:_____Total Carbs:_____

_____

_____

_____

Two Hour Glucose Reading:_____

Evening Snack:_____

Date:_____

A.M. Glucose Reading:_____

Breakfast:

Time:_____ Total Carbs:_____

_____

_____

_____

Two Hour Glucose Reading:_____

Mid Morning Snack:_____

Lunch:

Time:_____ Total Carbs:_____

_____

_____

_____

Two Hour Glucose Reading:_____

Mid Afternoon Snack:_____

Dinner:

Time:_____Total Carbs:_____

_____

_____

_____

Two Hour Glucose Reading:_____

Evening Snack:_____

Date:_____

A.M. Glucose Reading:_____

---

Breakfast:

Time:_____    Total Carbs:_____

_____
_____
_____

Two Hour Glucose Reading:_____
Mid Morning Snack:_____

---

Lunch:

Time:_____    Total Carbs:_____

_____
_____
_____

Two Hour Glucose Reading:_____
Mid Afternoon Snack:_____

---

Dinner:

Time:_____    Total Carbs:_____

_____
_____
_____

Two Hour Glucose Reading:_____
Evening Snack:_____

Date:_____

A.M. Glucose Reading:_____

Breakfast:

Time:_____ Total Carbs:_____
_____
_____
_____
Two Hour Glucose Reading:_____
Mid Morning Snack:_____

Lunch:

Time:_____ Total Carbs:_____
_____
_____
_____
Two Hour Glucose Reading:_____
Mid Afternoon Snack:_____

Dinner:

Time:_____Total Carbs:_____
_____
_____
_____
Two Hour Glucose Reading:_____
Evening Snack:_____

Date:_____

A.M. Glucose Reading:_____

Breakfast:

Time:_____  Total Carbs:_____

_____
_____
_____

Two Hour Glucose Reading:_____
Mid Morning Snack:_____

Lunch:

Time:_____  Total Carbs:_____

_____
_____
_____

Two Hour Glucose Reading:_____
Mid Afternoon Snack:_____

Dinner:

Time:_____Total Carbs:_____

_____
_____
_____

Two Hour Glucose Reading:_____
Evening Snack:_____

Date:_____

A.M. Glucose Reading:_____

Breakfast:

Time:_____  Total Carbs:_____
_____
_____
_____

Two Hour Glucose Reading:_____
Mid Morning Snack:_____

Lunch:

Time:_____  Total Carbs:_____
_____
_____
_____

Two Hour Glucose Reading:_____
Mid Afternoon Snack:_____

Dinner:

Time:_____Total Carbs:_____
_____
_____
_____

Two Hour Glucose Reading:_____
Evening Snack:_____

Date:_____

A.M. Glucose Reading:_____

Breakfast:

Time:_____  Total Carbs:_____
_____
_____
_____

Two Hour Glucose Reading:_____
Mid Morning Snack:_____

Lunch:

Time:_____  Total Carbs:_____
_____
_____
_____

Two Hour Glucose Reading:_____
Mid Afternoon Snack:_____

Dinner:

Time:_____Total Carbs:_____
_____
_____
_____

Two Hour Glucose Reading:_____
Evening Snack:_____

Date:_____

A.M. Glucose Reading:_____

Breakfast:

Time:_____  Total Carbs:_____

_____
_____
_____

Two Hour Glucose Reading:_____
Mid Morning Snack:_____

Lunch:

Time:_____  Total Carbs:_____

_____
_____
_____

Two Hour Glucose Reading:_____
Mid Afternoon Snack:_____

Dinner:

Time:_____Total Carbs:_____

_____
_____
_____

Two Hour Glucose Reading:_____
Evening Snack:_____

Date:_____

A.M. Glucose Reading:_____

---

Breakfast:

Time:_____ Total Carbs:_____

_____

_____

_____

Two Hour Glucose Reading:_____

Mid Morning Snack:_____

---

Lunch:

Time:_____ Total Carbs:_____

_____

_____

_____

Two Hour Glucose Reading:_____

Mid Afternoon Snack:_____

---

Dinner:

Time:_____Total Carbs:_____

_____

_____

_____

Two Hour Glucose Reading:_____

Evening Snack:_____

Date:_____

A.M. Glucose Reading:_____

Breakfast:

Time:_____ Total Carbs:_____

_____
_____
_____

Two Hour Glucose Reading:_____
Mid Morning Snack:_____

Lunch:

Time:_____ Total Carbs:_____

_____
_____
_____

Two Hour Glucose Reading:_____
Mid Afternoon Snack:_____

Dinner:

Time:_____Total Carbs:_____

_____
_____
_____

Two Hour Glucose Reading:_____
Evening Snack:_____

Date:_____

A.M. Glucose Reading:_____

---

Breakfast:

Time:_____ Total Carbs:_____

_____

_____

_____

Two Hour Glucose Reading:_____

Mid Morning Snack:_____

---

Lunch:

Time:_____ Total Carbs:_____

_____

_____

_____

Two Hour Glucose Reading:_____

Mid Afternoon Snack:_____

---

Dinner:

Time:_____Total Carbs:_____

_____

_____

_____

Two Hour Glucose Reading:_____

Evening Snack:_____

Date:_____

A.M. Glucose Reading:_____

Breakfast:

Time:_____ Total Carbs:_____

_____

_____

_____

Two Hour Glucose Reading:_____
Mid Morning Snack:_____

Lunch:

Time:_____ Total Carbs:_____

_____

_____

_____

Two Hour Glucose Reading:_____
Mid Afternoon Snack:_____

Dinner:

Time:_____Total Carbs:_____

_____

_____

_____

Two Hour Glucose Reading:_____
Evening Snack:_____

Date:_____

A.M. Glucose Reading:_____

Breakfast:

Time:_____  Total Carbs:_____
_____
_____
_____

Two Hour Glucose Reading:_____
Mid Morning Snack:_____

Lunch:

Time:_____  Total Carbs:_____
_____
_____
_____

Two Hour Glucose Reading:_____
Mid Afternoon Snack:_____

Dinner:

Time:_____Total Carbs:_____
_____
_____
_____

Two Hour Glucose Reading:_____
Evening Snack:_____

Date:_____

A.M. Glucose Reading:_____

Breakfast:

Time:_____ Total Carbs:_____

_____
_____
_____

Two Hour Glucose Reading:_____

Mid Morning Snack:_____

Lunch:

Time:_____ Total Carbs:_____

_____
_____
_____

Two Hour Glucose Reading:_____

Mid Afternoon Snack:_____

Dinner:

Time:_____Total Carbs:_____

_____
_____
_____

Two Hour Glucose Reading:_____

Evening Snack:_____

Date:_____

A.M. Glucose Reading:_____

Breakfast:

Time:_____ Total Carbs:_____

_____
_____
_____

Two Hour Glucose Reading:_____
Mid Morning Snack:_____

Lunch:

Time:_____ Total Carbs:_____

_____
_____
_____

Two Hour Glucose Reading:_____
Mid Afternoon Snack:_____

Dinner:

Time:_____Total Carbs:_____

_____
_____
_____

Two Hour Glucose Reading:_____
Evening Snack:_____

Date:_____

A.M. Glucose Reading:_____

Breakfast:

Time:_____    Total Carbs:_____

_____

_____

_____

Two Hour Glucose Reading:_____

Mid Morning Snack:_____

Lunch:

Time:_____    Total Carbs:_____

_____

_____

_____

Two Hour Glucose Reading:_____

Mid Afternoon Snack:_____

Dinner:

Time:_____Total Carbs:_____

_____

_____

_____

Two Hour Glucose Reading:_____

Evening Snack:_____

Date:_____

A.M. Glucose Reading:_____

---

Breakfast:

Time:_____    Total Carbs:_____

_____
_____
_____

Two Hour Glucose Reading:_____
Mid Morning Snack:_____

---

Lunch:

Time:_____    Total Carbs:_____

_____
_____
_____

Two Hour Glucose Reading:_____
Mid Afternoon Snack:_____

---

Dinner:

Time:_____    Total Carbs:_____

_____
_____
_____

Two Hour Glucose Reading:_____
Evening Snack:_____

Date:_____

A.M. Glucose Reading:_____

Breakfast:

Time:_____ Total Carbs:_____
_____
_____
_____

Two Hour Glucose Reading:_____
Mid Morning Snack:_____

Lunch:

Time:_____ Total Carbs:_____
_____
_____
_____

Two Hour Glucose Reading:_____
Mid Afternoon Snack:_____

Dinner:

Time:_____Total Carbs:_____
_____
_____
_____

Two Hour Glucose Reading:_____
Evening Snack:_____

Date:_____

A.M. Glucose Reading:_____

Breakfast:

Time:_____ Total Carbs:_____

_____

_____

_____

Two Hour Glucose Reading:_____

Mid Morning Snack:_____

Lunch:

Time:_____ Total Carbs:_____

_____

_____

_____

Two Hour Glucose Reading:_____

Mid Afternoon Snack:_____

Dinner:

Time:_____Total Carbs:_____

_____

_____

_____

Two Hour Glucose Reading:_____

Evening Snack:_____

Date:_____

A.M. Glucose Reading:_____

Breakfast:

Time:_____ Total Carbs:_____

_____

_____

_____

Two Hour Glucose Reading:_____

Mid Morning Snack:_____

---

Lunch:

Time:_____ Total Carbs:_____

_____

_____

_____

Two Hour Glucose Reading:_____

Mid Afternoon Snack:_____

---

Dinner:

Time:_____Total Carbs:_____

_____

_____

_____

Two Hour Glucose Reading:_____

Evening Snack:_____

Date:_____

A.M. Glucose Reading:_____

---

Breakfast:

Time:_____  Total Carbs:_____

_____
_____
_____

Two Hour Glucose Reading:_____
Mid Morning Snack:_____

---

Lunch:

Time:_____  Total Carbs:_____

_____
_____
_____

Two Hour Glucose Reading:_____
Mid Afternoon Snack:_____

---

Dinner:

Time:_____Total Carbs:_____

_____
_____
_____

Two Hour Glucose Reading:_____
Evening Snack:_____

Date:_____

A.M. Glucose Reading:_____

Breakfast:

Time:_____  Total Carbs:_____

_____

_____

_____

Two Hour Glucose Reading:_____

Mid Morning Snack:_____

Lunch:

Time:_____  Total Carbs:_____

_____

_____

_____

Two Hour Glucose Reading:_____

Mid Afternoon Snack:_____

Dinner:

Time:_____Total Carbs:_____

_____

_____

_____

Two Hour Glucose Reading:_____

Evening Snack:_____

Date:_____

A.M. Glucose Reading:_____

Breakfast:

Time:_____ Total Carbs:_____

_____

_____

_____

Two Hour Glucose Reading:_____

Mid Morning Snack:_____

Lunch:

Time:_____ Total Carbs:_____

_____

_____

_____

Two Hour Glucose Reading:_____

Mid Afternoon Snack:_____

Dinner:

Time:_____Total Carbs:_____

_____

_____

_____

Two Hour Glucose Reading:_____

Evening Snack:_____

Date:_____

A.M. Glucose Reading:_____

Breakfast:

Time:_____ Total Carbs:_____
_____
_____
_____

Two Hour Glucose Reading:_____
Mid Morning Snack:_____

Lunch:

Time:_____ Total Carbs:_____
_____
_____
_____

Two Hour Glucose Reading:_____
Mid Afternoon Snack:_____

Dinner:

Time:_____Total Carbs:_____
_____
_____
_____

Two Hour Glucose Reading:_____
Evening Snack:_____

Date:_____

A.M. Glucose Reading:_____

---

Breakfast:

Time:_____ Total Carbs:_____

_____
_____
_____

Two Hour Glucose Reading:_____
Mid Morning Snack:_____

---

Lunch:

Time:_____ Total Carbs:_____

_____
_____
_____

Two Hour Glucose Reading:_____
Mid Afternoon Snack:_____

---

Dinner:

Time:_____ Total Carbs:_____

_____
_____
_____

Two Hour Glucose Reading:_____
Evening Snack:_____

Date:_____

A.M. Glucose Reading:_____

Breakfast:

Time:_____ Total Carbs:_____

_____

_____

_____

Two Hour Glucose Reading:_____

Mid Morning Snack:_____

Lunch:

Time:_____ Total Carbs:_____

_____

_____

_____

Two Hour Glucose Reading:_____

Mid Afternoon Snack:_____

Dinner:

Time:_____ Total Carbs:_____

_____

_____

_____

Two Hour Glucose Reading:_____

Evening Snack:_____

Date:_____

A.M. Glucose Reading:_____

---

**Breakfast:**

Time:_____ Total Carbs:_____

_____

_____

_____

Two Hour Glucose Reading:_____

Mid Morning Snack:_____

---

**Lunch:**

Time:_____ Total Carbs:_____

_____

_____

_____

Two Hour Glucose Reading:_____

Mid Afternoon Snack:_____

---

**Dinner:**

Time:_____Total Carbs:_____

_____

_____

_____

Two Hour Glucose Reading:_____

Evening Snack:_____

Date:_____

A.M. Glucose Reading:_____

Breakfast:

Time:_____ Total Carbs:_____

_____
_____
_____

Two Hour Glucose Reading:_____
Mid Morning Snack:_____

Lunch:

Time:_____ Total Carbs:_____

_____
_____
_____

Two Hour Glucose Reading:_____
Mid Afternoon Snack:_____

Dinner:

Time:_____Total Carbs:_____

_____
_____
_____

Two Hour Glucose Reading:_____
Evening Snack:_____

Date:_____

A.M. Glucose Reading:_____

---

Breakfast:

Time:_____     Total Carbs:_____

_____

_____

_____

Two Hour Glucose Reading:_____

Mid Morning Snack:_____

---

Lunch:

Time:_____     Total Carbs:_____

_____

_____

_____

Two Hour Glucose Reading:_____

Mid Afternoon Snack:_____

---

Dinner:

Time:_____Total Carbs:_____

_____

_____

_____

Two Hour Glucose Reading:_____

Evening Snack:_____

Date:_____

A.M. Glucose Reading:_____

Breakfast:

Time:_____ Total Carbs:_____
_____
_____
_____

Two Hour Glucose Reading:_____
Mid Morning Snack:_____

Lunch:

Time:_____ Total Carbs:_____
_____
_____
_____

Two Hour Glucose Reading:_____
Mid Afternoon Snack:_____

Dinner:

Time:_____Total Carbs:_____
_____
_____
_____

Two Hour Glucose Reading:_____
Evening Snack:_____

Date:_____

A.M. Glucose Reading:_____

Breakfast:

Time:_____ Total Carbs:_____

_____
_____
_____

Two Hour Glucose Reading:_____
Mid Morning Snack:_____

Lunch:

Time:_____ Total Carbs:_____

_____
_____
_____

Two Hour Glucose Reading:_____
Mid Afternoon Snack:_____

Dinner:

Time:_____Total Carbs:_____

_____
_____
_____

Two Hour Glucose Reading:_____
Evening Snack:_____

Date:_____

A.M. Glucose Reading:_____

Breakfast:

Time:_____ Total Carbs:_____

_____

_____

_____

Two Hour Glucose Reading:_____

Mid Morning Snack:_____

Lunch:

Time:_____ Total Carbs:_____

_____

_____

_____

Two Hour Glucose Reading:_____

Mid Afternoon Snack:_____

Dinner:

Time:_____Total Carbs:_____

_____

_____

_____

Two Hour Glucose Reading:_____

Evening Snack:_____

Date:_____

A.M. Glucose Reading:_____

Breakfast:

Time:_____   Total Carbs:_____

_____

_____

_____

Two Hour Glucose Reading:_____

Mid Morning Snack:_____

Lunch:

Time:_____   Total Carbs:_____

_____

_____

_____

Two Hour Glucose Reading:_____

Mid Afternoon Snack:_____

Dinner:

Time:_____Total Carbs:_____

_____

_____

_____

Two Hour Glucose Reading:_____

Evening Snack:_____

Date:_____

A.M. Glucose Reading:_____

Breakfast:

Time:_____ Total Carbs:_____

_____
_____
_____

Two Hour Glucose Reading:_____
Mid Morning Snack:_____

Lunch:

Time:_____ Total Carbs:_____

_____
_____
_____

Two Hour Glucose Reading:_____
Mid Afternoon Snack:_____

Dinner:

Time:_____Total Carbs:_____

_____
_____
_____

Two Hour Glucose Reading:_____
Evening Snack:_____

Date:_____

A.M. Glucose Reading:_____

Breakfast:

Time:_____    Total Carbs:_____

_____
_____
_____

Two Hour Glucose Reading:_____
Mid Morning Snack:_____

Lunch:

Time:_____    Total Carbs:_____

_____
_____
_____

Two Hour Glucose Reading:_____
Mid Afternoon Snack:_____

Dinner:

Time:_____Total Carbs:_____

_____
_____
_____

Two Hour Glucose Reading:_____
Evening Snack:_____

Date:_____

A.M. Glucose Reading:_____

Breakfast:

Time:_____ Total Carbs:_____
_____
_____
_____

Two Hour Glucose Reading:_____
Mid Morning Snack:_____

Lunch:

Time:_____ Total Carbs:_____
_____
_____
_____

Two Hour Glucose Reading:_____
Mid Afternoon Snack:_____

Dinner:

Time:_____Total Carbs:_____
_____
_____
_____

Two Hour Glucose Reading:_____
Evening Snack:_____

Date:_____

A.M. Glucose Reading:_____

---

Breakfast:

Time:_____    Total Carbs:_____

_____

_____

_____

Two Hour Glucose Reading:_____

Mid Morning Snack:_____

---

Lunch:

Time:_____    Total Carbs:_____

_____

_____

_____

Two Hour Glucose Reading:_____

Mid Afternoon Snack:_____

---

Dinner:

Time:_____Total Carbs:_____

_____

_____

_____

Two Hour Glucose Reading:_____

Evening Snack:_____

Date:_____

A.M. Glucose Reading:_____

Breakfast:

Time:_____ Total Carbs:_____
_____
_____
_____

Two Hour Glucose Reading:_____
Mid Morning Snack:_____

Lunch:

Time:_____ Total Carbs:_____
_____
_____
_____

Two Hour Glucose Reading:_____
Mid Afternoon Snack:_____

Dinner:

Time:_____Total Carbs:_____
_____
_____
_____

Two Hour Glucose Reading:_____
Evening Snack:_____

Date:_____

A.M. Glucose Reading:_____

---

Breakfast:

Time:_____ Total Carbs:_____

_____

_____

_____

Two Hour Glucose Reading:_____

Mid Morning Snack:_____

---

Lunch:

Time:_____ Total Carbs:_____

_____

_____

_____

Two Hour Glucose Reading:_____

Mid Afternoon Snack:_____

---

Dinner:

Time:_____Total Carbs:_____

_____

_____

_____

Two Hour Glucose Reading:_____

Evening Snack:_____

Date:_____

A.M. Glucose Reading:_____

Breakfast:

Time:_____ Total Carbs:_____

_____

_____

_____

Two Hour Glucose Reading:_____

Mid Morning Snack:_____

Lunch:

Time:_____ Total Carbs:_____

_____

_____

_____

Two Hour Glucose Reading:_____

Mid Afternoon Snack:_____

Dinner:

Time:_____Total Carbs:_____

_____

_____

_____

Two Hour Glucose Reading:_____

Evening Snack:_____

Date:_____

A.M. Glucose Reading:_____

Breakfast:

Time:_____     Total Carbs:_____

_____

_____

_____

Two Hour Glucose Reading:_____

Mid Morning Snack:_____

Lunch:

Time:_____     Total Carbs:_____

_____

_____

_____

Two Hour Glucose Reading:_____

Mid Afternoon Snack:_____

Dinner:

Time:_____Total Carbs:_____

_____

_____

_____

Two Hour Glucose Reading:_____

Evening Snack:_____

Date:_____

A.M. Glucose Reading:_____

---

**Breakfast:**

Time:_____    Total Carbs:_____
_____
_____
_____

Two Hour Glucose Reading:_____
Mid Morning Snack:_____

---

**Lunch:**

Time:_____    Total Carbs:_____
_____
_____
_____

Two Hour Glucose Reading:_____
Mid Afternoon Snack:_____

---

**Dinner:**

Time:_____Total Carbs:_____
_____
_____
_____

Two Hour Glucose Reading:_____
Evening Snack:_____

Date:_____

A.M. Glucose Reading:_____

Breakfast:

Time:_____  Total Carbs:_____

_____
_____
_____

Two Hour Glucose Reading:_____
Mid Morning Snack:_____

Lunch:

Time:_____  Total Carbs:_____

_____
_____
_____

Two Hour Glucose Reading:_____
Mid Afternoon Snack:_____

Dinner:

Time:_____Total Carbs:_____

_____
_____
_____

Two Hour Glucose Reading:_____
Evening Snack:_____

Date:_____

A.M. Glucose Reading:_____

Breakfast:

Time:_____  Total Carbs:_____

_____

_____

_____

Two Hour Glucose Reading:_____

Mid Morning Snack:_____

Lunch:

Time:_____  Total Carbs:_____

_____

_____

_____

Two Hour Glucose Reading:_____

Mid Afternoon Snack:_____

Dinner:

Time:_____Total Carbs:_____

_____

_____

_____

Two Hour Glucose Reading:_____

Evening Snack:_____

Date:_____

A.M. Glucose Reading:_____

Breakfast:

Time:_____     Total Carbs:_____

_____

_____

_____

Two Hour Glucose Reading:_____

Mid Morning Snack:_____

Lunch:

Time:_____     Total Carbs:_____

_____

_____

_____

Two Hour Glucose Reading:_____

Mid Afternoon Snack:_____

Dinner:

Time:_____     Total Carbs:_____

_____

_____

_____

Two Hour Glucose Reading:_____

Evening Snack:_____

Date:_____

A.M. Glucose Reading:_____

Breakfast:

Time:_____ Total Carbs:_____

_____
_____
_____

Two Hour Glucose Reading:_____
Mid Morning Snack:_____

Lunch:

Time:_____ Total Carbs:_____

_____
_____
_____

Two Hour Glucose Reading:_____
Mid Afternoon Snack:_____

Dinner:

Time:_____Total Carbs:_____

_____
_____
_____

Two Hour Glucose Reading:_____
Evening Snack:_____

Date:_____

A.M. Glucose Reading:_____

Breakfast:

Time:_____    Total Carbs:_____

_____
_____
_____

Two Hour Glucose Reading:_____
Mid Morning Snack:_____

Lunch:

Time:_____    Total Carbs:_____

_____
_____
_____

Two Hour Glucose Reading:_____
Mid Afternoon Snack:_____

Dinner:

Time:_____Total Carbs:_____

_____
_____
_____

Two Hour Glucose Reading:_____
Evening Snack:_____

Date:_____

A.M. Glucose Reading:_____

---

Breakfast:

Time:_____  Total Carbs:_____

_____
_____
_____

Two Hour Glucose Reading:_____
Mid Morning Snack:_____

---

Lunch:

Time:_____  Total Carbs:_____

_____
_____
_____

Two Hour Glucose Reading:_____
Mid Afternoon Snack:_____

---

Dinner:

Time:_____Total Carbs:_____

_____
_____
_____

Two Hour Glucose Reading:_____
Evening Snack:_____

Date:_____

A.M. Glucose Reading:_____

Breakfast:

Time:_____ Total Carbs:_____

_____

_____

_____

Two Hour Glucose Reading:_____

Mid Morning Snack:_____

Lunch:

Time:_____ Total Carbs:_____

_____

_____

_____

Two Hour Glucose Reading:_____

Mid Afternoon Snack:_____

Dinner:

Time:_____Total Carbs:_____

_____

_____

_____

Two Hour Glucose Reading:_____

Evening Snack:_____

Date:_____

A.M. Glucose Reading:_____

Breakfast:

Time:_____ Total Carbs:_____

_____
_____
_____

Two Hour Glucose Reading:_____

Mid Morning Snack:_____

Lunch:

Time:_____ Total Carbs:_____

_____
_____
_____

Two Hour Glucose Reading:_____

Mid Afternoon Snack:_____

Dinner:

Time:_____Total Carbs:_____

_____
_____
_____

Two Hour Glucose Reading:_____

Evening Snack:_____

Date:_____

A.M. Glucose Reading:_____

Breakfast:

Time:_____ Total Carbs:_____

_____
_____
_____

Two Hour Glucose Reading:_____
Mid Morning Snack:_____

Lunch:

Time:_____ Total Carbs:_____

_____
_____
_____

Two Hour Glucose Reading:_____
Mid Afternoon Snack:_____

Dinner:

Time:_____Total Carbs:_____

_____
_____
_____

Two Hour Glucose Reading:_____
Evening Snack:_____

Date:_____

A.M. Glucose Reading:_____

Breakfast:

Time:_____ Total Carbs:_____
_____
_____
_____

Two Hour Glucose Reading:_____
Mid Morning Snack:_____

Lunch:

Time:_____ Total Carbs:_____
_____
_____
_____

Two Hour Glucose Reading:_____
Mid Afternoon Snack:_____

Dinner:

Time:_____Total Carbs:_____
_____
_____
_____

Two Hour Glucose Reading:_____
Evening Snack:_____

Date:_____

A.M. Glucose Reading:_____

Breakfast:

Time:_____   Total Carbs:_____

_____
_____
_____

Two Hour Glucose Reading:_____
Mid Morning Snack:_____

Lunch:

Time:_____   Total Carbs:_____

_____
_____
_____

Two Hour Glucose Reading:_____
Mid Afternoon Snack:_____

Dinner:

Time:_____Total Carbs:_____

_____
_____
_____

Two Hour Glucose Reading:_____
Evening Snack:_____

Date:_____

A.M. Glucose Reading:_____

---

Breakfast:

Time:_____ Total Carbs:_____

_____

_____

_____

Two Hour Glucose Reading:_____

Mid Morning Snack:_____

---

Lunch:

Time:_____ Total Carbs:_____

_____

_____

_____

Two Hour Glucose Reading:_____

Mid Afternoon Snack:_____

---

Dinner:

Time:_____Total Carbs:_____

_____

_____

_____

Two Hour Glucose Reading:_____

Evening Snack:_____

Date:_____

A.M. Glucose Reading:_____

Breakfast:

Time:_____    Total Carbs:_____

_____

_____

_____

Two Hour Glucose Reading:_____
Mid Morning Snack:_____

Lunch:

Time:_____    Total Carbs:_____

_____

_____

_____

Two Hour Glucose Reading:_____
Mid Afternoon Snack:_____

Dinner:

Time:_____Total Carbs:_____

_____

_____

_____

Two Hour Glucose Reading:_____
Evening Snack:_____

Date:_____

A.M. Glucose Reading:_____

---

Breakfast:

Time:_____ Total Carbs:_____

_____

_____

_____

Two Hour Glucose Reading:_____

Mid Morning Snack:_____

---

Lunch:

Time:_____ Total Carbs:_____

_____

_____

_____

Two Hour Glucose Reading:_____

Mid Afternoon Snack:_____

---

Dinner:

Time:_____Total Carbs:_____

_____

_____

_____

Two Hour Glucose Reading:_____

Evening Snack:_____

Date:_____

A.M. Glucose Reading:_____

---

Breakfast:

Time:_____  Total Carbs:_____

_____
_____
_____

Two Hour Glucose Reading:_____
Mid Morning Snack:_____

---

Lunch:

Time:_____  Total Carbs:_____

_____
_____
_____

Two Hour Glucose Reading:_____
Mid Afternoon Snack:_____

---

Dinner:

Time:_____Total Carbs:_____

_____
_____
_____

Two Hour Glucose Reading:_____
Evening Snack:_____

Date:_____

A.M. Glucose Reading:_____

Breakfast:

Time:_____  Total Carbs:_____

_____

_____

_____

Two Hour Glucose Reading:_____

Mid Morning Snack:_____

Lunch:

Time:_____  Total Carbs:_____

_____

_____

_____

Two Hour Glucose Reading:_____

Mid Afternoon Snack:_____

Dinner:

Time:_____Total Carbs:_____

_____

_____

_____

Two Hour Glucose Reading:_____

Evening Snack:_____

Date:_____

A.M. Glucose Reading:_____

Breakfast:

Time:_____ Total Carbs:_____

_____

_____

_____

Two Hour Glucose Reading:_____

Mid Morning Snack:_____

Lunch:

Time:_____ Total Carbs:_____

_____

_____

_____

Two Hour Glucose Reading:_____

Mid Afternoon Snack:_____

Dinner:

Time:_____Total Carbs:_____

_____

_____

_____

Two Hour Glucose Reading:_____

Evening Snack:_____

Date:_____

A.M. Glucose Reading:_____

Breakfast:

Time:_____ Total Carbs:_____

_____
_____
_____

Two Hour Glucose Reading:_____
Mid Morning Snack:_____

Lunch:

Time:_____ Total Carbs:_____

_____
_____
_____

Two Hour Glucose Reading:_____
Mid Afternoon Snack:_____

Dinner:

Time:_____Total Carbs:_____

_____
_____
_____

Two Hour Glucose Reading:_____
Evening Snack:_____

Date:_____

A.M. Glucose Reading:_____

Breakfast:

Time:_____ Total Carbs:_____
_____
_____
_____

Two Hour Glucose Reading:_____
Mid Morning Snack:_____

Lunch:

Time:_____ Total Carbs:_____
_____
_____
_____

Two Hour Glucose Reading:_____
Mid Afternoon Snack:_____

Dinner:

Time:_____Total Carbs:_____
_____
_____
_____

Two Hour Glucose Reading:_____
Evening Snack:_____

Date:_____

A.M. Glucose Reading:_____

Breakfast:

Time:_____ Total Carbs:_____

_____
_____
_____

Two Hour Glucose Reading:_____
Mid Morning Snack:_____

Lunch:

Time:_____ Total Carbs:_____

_____
_____
_____

Two Hour Glucose Reading:_____
Mid Afternoon Snack:_____

Dinner:

Time:_____Total Carbs:_____

_____
_____
_____

Two Hour Glucose Reading:_____
Evening Snack:_____

Date:_____

A.M. Glucose Reading:_____

Breakfast:

Time:_____ Total Carbs:_____

_____
_____
_____

Two Hour Glucose Reading:_____
Mid Morning Snack:_____

Lunch:

Time:_____ Total Carbs:_____

_____
_____
_____

Two Hour Glucose Reading:_____
Mid Afternoon Snack:_____

Dinner:

Time:_____Total Carbs:_____

_____
_____
_____

Two Hour Glucose Reading:_____
Evening Snack:_____

Date:_____

A.M. Glucose Reading:_____

---

Breakfast:

Time:_____ Total Carbs:_____
_____
_____
_____

Two Hour Glucose Reading:_____
Mid Morning Snack:_____

---

Lunch:

Time:_____ Total Carbs:_____
_____
_____
_____

Two Hour Glucose Reading:_____
Mid Afternoon Snack:_____

---

Dinner:

Time:_____Total Carbs:_____
_____
_____
_____

Two Hour Glucose Reading:_____
Evening Snack:_____

Date:_____

A.M. Glucose Reading:_____

Breakfast:

Time:_____ Total Carbs:_____

_____

_____

_____

Two Hour Glucose Reading:_____

Mid Morning Snack:_____

Lunch:

Time:_____ Total Carbs:_____

_____

_____

_____

Two Hour Glucose Reading:_____

Mid Afternoon Snack:_____

Dinner:

Time:_____Total Carbs:_____

_____

_____

_____

Two Hour Glucose Reading:_____

Evening Snack:_____

Date:_____

A.M. Glucose Reading:_____

Breakfast:

Time:_____ Total Carbs:_____
_____
_____
_____

Two Hour Glucose Reading:_____
Mid Morning Snack:_____

Lunch:

Time:_____ Total Carbs:_____
_____
_____
_____

Two Hour Glucose Reading:_____
Mid Afternoon Snack:_____

Dinner:

Time:_____Total Carbs:_____
_____
_____
_____

Two Hour Glucose Reading:_____
Evening Snack:_____

Date:_____

A.M. Glucose Reading:_____

Breakfast:

Time:_____ Total Carbs:_____

_____
_____
_____

Two Hour Glucose Reading:_____
Mid Morning Snack:_____

Lunch:

Time:_____ Total Carbs:_____

_____
_____
_____

Two Hour Glucose Reading:_____
Mid Afternoon Snack:_____

Dinner:

Time:_____Total Carbs:_____

_____
_____
_____

Two Hour Glucose Reading:_____
Evening Snack:_____

Date:_____

A.M. Glucose Reading:_____

Breakfast:

Time:_____ Total Carbs:_____
_____
_____
_____

Two Hour Glucose Reading:_____
Mid Morning Snack:_____

Lunch:

Time:_____ Total Carbs:_____
_____
_____
_____

Two Hour Glucose Reading:_____
Mid Afternoon Snack:_____

Dinner:

Time:_____Total Carbs:_____
_____
_____
_____

Two Hour Glucose Reading:_____
Evening Snack:_____

Date:_____

A.M. Glucose Reading:_____

Breakfast:

Time:_____ Total Carbs:_____

_____
_____
_____

Two Hour Glucose Reading:_____
Mid Morning Snack:_____

Lunch:

Time:_____ Total Carbs:_____

_____
_____
_____

Two Hour Glucose Reading:_____
Mid Afternoon Snack:_____

Dinner:

Time:_____Total Carbs:_____

_____
_____
_____

Two Hour Glucose Reading:_____
Evening Snack:_____

Date:_____

A.M. Glucose Reading:_____

---

Breakfast:

Time:_____    Total Carbs:_____

_____
_____
_____

Two Hour Glucose Reading:_____
Mid Morning Snack:_____

---

Lunch:

Time:_____    Total Carbs:_____

_____
_____
_____

Two Hour Glucose Reading:_____
Mid Afternoon Snack:_____

---

Dinner:

Time:_____Total Carbs:_____

_____
_____
_____

Two Hour Glucose Reading:_____
Evening Snack:_____

Date:_____

A.M. Glucose Reading:_____

Breakfast:

Time:_____ Total Carbs:_____

_____
_____
_____

Two Hour Glucose Reading:_____
Mid Morning Snack:_____

Lunch:

Time:_____ Total Carbs:_____

_____
_____
_____

Two Hour Glucose Reading:_____
Mid Afternoon Snack:_____

Dinner:

Time:_____Total Carbs:_____

_____
_____
_____

Two Hour Glucose Reading:_____
Evening Snack:_____

Date:_____

A.M. Glucose Reading:_____

---

Breakfast:

Time:_____ Total Carbs:_____

_____

_____

_____

Two Hour Glucose Reading:_____

Mid Morning Snack:_____

---

Lunch:

Time:_____ Total Carbs:_____

_____

_____

_____

Two Hour Glucose Reading:_____

Mid Afternoon Snack:_____

---

Dinner:

Time:_____Total Carbs:_____

_____

_____

_____

Two Hour Glucose Reading:_____

Evening Snack:_____

Date:_____

A.M. Glucose Reading:_____

Breakfast:

Time:_____ Total Carbs:_____

_____

_____

_____

Two Hour Glucose Reading:_____

Mid Morning Snack:_____

Lunch:

Time:_____ Total Carbs:_____

_____

_____

_____

Two Hour Glucose Reading:_____

Mid Afternoon Snack:_____

Dinner:

Time:_____Total Carbs:_____

_____

_____

_____

Two Hour Glucose Reading:_____

Evening Snack:_____

Date:_____

A.M. Glucose Reading:_____

---

Breakfast:

Time:_____    Total Carbs:_____
_____
_____
_____

Two Hour Glucose Reading:_____
Mid Morning Snack:_____

---

Lunch:

Time:_____    Total Carbs:_____
_____
_____
_____

Two Hour Glucose Reading:_____
Mid Afternoon Snack:_____

---

Dinner:

Time:_____Total Carbs:_____
_____
_____
_____

Two Hour Glucose Reading:_____
Evening Snack:_____

Date:_____

A.M. Glucose Reading:_____

Breakfast:

Time:_____  Total Carbs:_____

_____

_____

_____

Two Hour Glucose Reading:_____
Mid Morning Snack:_____

Lunch:

Time:_____  Total Carbs:_____

_____

_____

_____

Two Hour Glucose Reading:_____
Mid Afternoon Snack:_____

Dinner:

Time:_____Total Carbs:_____

_____

_____

_____

Two Hour Glucose Reading:_____
Evening Snack:_____

Date:_____

A.M. Glucose Reading:_____

Breakfast:

Time:_____  Total Carbs:_____

_____

_____

_____

Two Hour Glucose Reading:_____

Mid Morning Snack:_____

Lunch:

Time:_____  Total Carbs:_____

_____

_____

_____

Two Hour Glucose Reading:_____

Mid Afternoon Snack:_____

Dinner:

Time:_____Total Carbs:_____

_____

_____

_____

Two Hour Glucose Reading:_____

Evening Snack:_____

Date:_____

A.M. Glucose Reading:_____

Breakfast:

Time:_____ Total Carbs:_____
_____
_____
_____

Two Hour Glucose Reading:_____
Mid Morning Snack:_____

Lunch:

Time:_____ Total Carbs:_____
_____
_____
_____

Two Hour Glucose Reading:_____
Mid Afternoon Snack:_____

Dinner:

Time:_____Total Carbs:_____
_____
_____
_____

Two Hour Glucose Reading:_____
Evening Snack:_____

Date:_____

A.M. Glucose Reading:_____

Breakfast:

Time:_____ Total Carbs:_____

_____

_____

_____

Two Hour Glucose Reading:_____

Mid Morning Snack:_____

Lunch:

Time:_____ Total Carbs:_____

_____

_____

_____

Two Hour Glucose Reading:_____

Mid Afternoon Snack:_____

Dinner:

Time:_____Total Carbs:_____

_____

_____

_____

Two Hour Glucose Reading:_____

Evening Snack:_____

Date:_____

A.M. Glucose Reading:_____

Breakfast:

Time:_____ Total Carbs:_____

_____

_____

_____

Two Hour Glucose Reading:_____

Mid Morning Snack:_____

Lunch:

Time:_____ Total Carbs:_____

_____

_____

_____

Two Hour Glucose Reading:_____

Mid Afternoon Snack:_____

Dinner:

Time:_____Total Carbs:_____

_____

_____

_____

Two Hour Glucose Reading:_____

Evening Snack:_____

Date:_____

A.M. Glucose Reading:_____

Breakfast:

Time:_____ Total Carbs:_____
_____
_____
_____

Two Hour Glucose Reading:_____
Mid Morning Snack:_____

Lunch:

Time:_____ Total Carbs:_____
_____
_____
_____

Two Hour Glucose Reading:_____
Mid Afternoon Snack:_____

Dinner:

Time:_____Total Carbs:_____
_____
_____
_____

Two Hour Glucose Reading:_____
Evening Snack:_____

Date:_____

A.M. Glucose Reading:_____

---

Breakfast:

Time:_____    Total Carbs:_____
_____
_____
_____

Two Hour Glucose Reading:_____
Mid Morning Snack:_____

---

Lunch:

Time:_____    Total Carbs:_____
_____
_____
_____

Two Hour Glucose Reading:_____
Mid Afternoon Snack:_____

---

Dinner:

Time:_____    Total Carbs:_____
_____
_____
_____

Two Hour Glucose Reading:_____
Evening Snack:_____

Date:_____

A.M. Glucose Reading:_____

Breakfast:

Time:_____ Total Carbs:_____

_____
_____
_____

Two Hour Glucose Reading:_____
Mid Morning Snack:_____

Lunch:

Time:_____ Total Carbs:_____

_____
_____
_____

Two Hour Glucose Reading:_____
Mid Afternoon Snack:_____

Dinner:

Time:_____Total Carbs:_____

_____
_____
_____

Two Hour Glucose Reading:_____
Evening Snack:_____

Date:_____

A.M. Glucose Reading:_____

Breakfast:

Time:_____ Total Carbs:_____
_____
_____
_____
Two Hour Glucose Reading:_____
Mid Morning Snack:_____

Lunch:

Time:_____ Total Carbs:_____
_____
_____
_____
Two Hour Glucose Reading:_____
Mid Afternoon Snack:_____

Dinner:

Time:_____Total Carbs:_____
_____
_____
_____
Two Hour Glucose Reading:_____
Evening Snack:_____

Date:_____

A.M. Glucose Reading:_____

---

Breakfast:

Time:_____  Total Carbs:_____

_____
_____
_____

Two Hour Glucose Reading:_____
Mid Morning Snack:_____

---

Lunch:

Time:_____  Total Carbs:_____

_____
_____
_____

Two Hour Glucose Reading:_____
Mid Afternoon Snack:_____

---

Dinner:

Time:_____Total Carbs:_____

_____
_____
_____

Two Hour Glucose Reading:_____
Evening Snack:_____

Date:_____

A.M. Glucose Reading:_____

Breakfast:

Time:_____ Total Carbs:_____

_____
_____
_____

Two Hour Glucose Reading:_____
Mid Morning Snack:_____

Lunch:

Time:_____ Total Carbs:_____

_____
_____
_____

Two Hour Glucose Reading:_____
Mid Afternoon Snack:_____

Dinner:

Time:_____Total Carbs:_____

_____
_____
_____

Two Hour Glucose Reading:_____
Evening Snack:_____

Date:_____

A.M. Glucose Reading:_____

---

Breakfast:

Time:_____ Total Carbs:_____

_____
_____
_____

Two Hour Glucose Reading:_____
Mid Morning Snack:_____

---

Lunch:

Time:_____ Total Carbs:_____

_____
_____
_____

Two Hour Glucose Reading:_____
Mid Afternoon Snack:_____

---

Dinner:

Time:_____Total Carbs:_____

_____
_____
_____

Two Hour Glucose Reading:_____
Evening Snack:_____

Date:_____

A.M. Glucose Reading:_____

Breakfast:

Time:_____ Total Carbs:_____
_____
_____
_____

Two Hour Glucose Reading:_____
Mid Morning Snack:_____

Lunch:

Time:_____ Total Carbs:_____
_____
_____
_____

Two Hour Glucose Reading:_____
Mid Afternoon Snack:_____

Dinner:

Time:_____Total Carbs:_____
_____
_____
_____

Two Hour Glucose Reading:_____
Evening Snack:_____

Date:_____

A.M. Glucose Reading:_____

Breakfast:

Time:_____ Total Carbs:_____
_____
_____
_____

Two Hour Glucose Reading:_____
Mid Morning Snack:_____

Lunch:

Time:_____ Total Carbs:_____
_____
_____
_____

Two Hour Glucose Reading:_____
Mid Afternoon Snack:_____

Dinner:

Time:_____Total Carbs:_____
_____
_____
_____

Two Hour Glucose Reading:_____
Evening Snack:_____

Date:_____

A.M. Glucose Reading:_____

Breakfast:

Time:_____ Total Carbs:_____

_____

_____

_____

Two Hour Glucose Reading:_____

Mid Morning Snack:_____

Lunch:

Time:_____ Total Carbs:_____

_____

_____

_____

Two Hour Glucose Reading:_____

Mid Afternoon Snack:_____

Dinner:

Time:_____Total Carbs:_____

_____

_____

_____

Two Hour Glucose Reading:_____

Evening Snack:_____

Date:_____

A.M. Glucose Reading:_____

---

Breakfast:

Time:_____ Total Carbs:_____

_____
_____
_____

Two Hour Glucose Reading:_____
Mid Morning Snack:_____

---

Lunch:

Time:_____ Total Carbs:_____

_____
_____
_____

Two Hour Glucose Reading:_____
Mid Afternoon Snack:_____

---

Dinner:

Time:_____Total Carbs:_____

_____
_____
_____

Two Hour Glucose Reading:_____
Evening Snack:_____

Date:_____

A.M. Glucose Reading:_____

Breakfast:

Time:_____ Total Carbs:_____

_____
_____
_____

Two Hour Glucose Reading:_____
Mid Morning Snack:_____

Lunch:

Time:_____ Total Carbs:_____

_____
_____
_____

Two Hour Glucose Reading:_____
Mid Afternoon Snack:_____

Dinner:

Time:_____Total Carbs:_____

_____
_____
_____

Two Hour Glucose Reading:_____
Evening Snack:_____

Date:_____

A.M. Glucose Reading:_____

Breakfast:

Time:_____ Total Carbs:_____

_____

_____

_____

Two Hour Glucose Reading:_____

Mid Morning Snack:_____

Lunch:

Time:_____ Total Carbs:_____

_____

_____

_____

Two Hour Glucose Reading:_____

Mid Afternoon Snack:_____

Dinner:

Time:_____Total Carbs:_____

_____

_____

_____

Two Hour Glucose Reading:_____

Evening Snack:_____

Date:_____

A.M. Glucose Reading:_____

Breakfast:

Time:_____ Total Carbs:_____

_____
_____
_____

Two Hour Glucose Reading:_____
Mid Morning Snack:_____

Lunch:

Time:_____ Total Carbs:_____

_____
_____
_____

Two Hour Glucose Reading:_____
Mid Afternoon Snack:_____

Dinner:

Time:_____Total Carbs:_____

_____
_____
_____

Two Hour Glucose Reading:_____
Evening Snack:_____

Date:_____

A.M. Glucose Reading:_____

---

Breakfast:

Time:_____  Total Carbs:_____

_____
_____
_____

Two Hour Glucose Reading:_____
Mid Morning Snack:_____

---

Lunch:

Time:_____  Total Carbs:_____

_____
_____
_____

Two Hour Glucose Reading:_____
Mid Afternoon Snack:_____

---

Dinner:

Time:_____Total Carbs:_____

_____
_____
_____

Two Hour Glucose Reading:_____
Evening Snack:_____

Date:_____

A.M. Glucose Reading:_____

---

Breakfast:

Time:_____ Total Carbs:_____

_____

_____

_____

Two Hour Glucose Reading:_____

Mid Morning Snack:_____

---

Lunch:

Time:_____ Total Carbs:_____

_____

_____

_____

Two Hour Glucose Reading:_____

Mid Afternoon Snack:_____

---

Dinner:

Time:_____ Total Carbs:_____

_____

_____

_____

Two Hour Glucose Reading:_____

Evening Snack:_____

Date:_____

A.M. Glucose Reading:_____

Breakfast:

Time:_____ Total Carbs:_____

_____

_____

_____

Two Hour Glucose Reading:_____

Mid Morning Snack:_____

Lunch:

Time:_____ Total Carbs:_____

_____

_____

_____

Two Hour Glucose Reading:_____

Mid Afternoon Snack:_____

Dinner:

Time:_____Total Carbs:_____

_____

_____

_____

Two Hour Glucose Reading:_____

Evening Snack:_____

Date:_____

A.M. Glucose Reading:_____

Breakfast:

Time:_____ Total Carbs:_____

_____
_____
_____

Two Hour Glucose Reading:_____
Mid Morning Snack:_____

Lunch:

Time:_____ Total Carbs:_____

_____
_____
_____

Two Hour Glucose Reading:_____
Mid Afternoon Snack:_____

Dinner:

Time:_____Total Carbs:_____

_____
_____
_____

Two Hour Glucose Reading:_____
Evening Snack:_____

Date:_____

A.M. Glucose Reading:_____

Breakfast:

Time:_____ Total Carbs:_____
_____
_____
_____

Two Hour Glucose Reading:_____
Mid Morning Snack:_____

Lunch:

Time:_____ Total Carbs:_____
_____
_____
_____

Two Hour Glucose Reading:_____
Mid Afternoon Snack:_____

Dinner:

Time:_____Total Carbs:_____
_____
_____
_____

Two Hour Glucose Reading:_____
Evening Snack:_____

Date:_____

A.M. Glucose Reading:_____

Breakfast:

Time:_____ Total Carbs:_____

_____
_____
_____

Two Hour Glucose Reading:_____
Mid Morning Snack:_____

Lunch:

Time:_____ Total Carbs:_____

_____
_____
_____

Two Hour Glucose Reading:_____
Mid Afternoon Snack:_____

Dinner:

Time:_____Total Carbs:_____

_____
_____
_____

Two Hour Glucose Reading:_____
Evening Snack:_____

Date:_____

A.M. Glucose Reading:_____

Breakfast:

Time:_____  Total Carbs:_____

_____

_____

_____

Two Hour Glucose Reading:_____

Mid Morning Snack:_____

Lunch:

Time:_____  Total Carbs:_____

_____

_____

_____

Two Hour Glucose Reading:_____

Mid Afternoon Snack:_____

Dinner:

Time:_____Total Carbs:_____

_____

_____

_____

Two Hour Glucose Reading:_____

Evening Snack:_____

Date:_____

A.M. Glucose Reading:_____

Breakfast:

Time:_____    Total Carbs:_____

_____

_____

_____

Two Hour Glucose Reading:_____

Mid Morning Snack:_____

Lunch:

Time:_____    Total Carbs:_____

_____

_____

_____

Two Hour Glucose Reading:_____
Mid Afternoon Snack:_____

Dinner:

Time:_____    Total Carbs:_____

_____

_____

_____

Two Hour Glucose Reading:_____
Evening Snack:_____

Date:_____

A.M. Glucose Reading:_____

---

Breakfast:

Time:_____    Total Carbs:_____

_____

_____

_____

Two Hour Glucose Reading:_____

Mid Morning Snack:_____

---

Lunch:

Time:_____    Total Carbs:_____

_____

_____

_____

Two Hour Glucose Reading:_____

Mid Afternoon Snack:_____

---

Dinner:

Time:_____Total Carbs:_____

_____

_____

_____

Two Hour Glucose Reading:_____

Evening Snack:_____

Date:_____

A.M. Glucose Reading:_____

Breakfast:

Time:_____    Total Carbs:_____
_____
_____
_____

Two Hour Glucose Reading:_____
Mid Morning Snack:_____

Lunch:

Time:_____    Total Carbs:_____
_____
_____
_____

Two Hour Glucose Reading:_____
Mid Afternoon Snack:_____

Dinner:

Time:_____Total Carbs:_____
_____
_____
_____

Two Hour Glucose Reading:_____
Evening Snack:_____

Date:_____

A.M. Glucose Reading:_____

Breakfast:

Time:_____ Total Carbs:_____

_____

_____

_____

Two Hour Glucose Reading:_____

Mid Morning Snack:_____

Lunch:

Time:_____ Total Carbs:_____

_____

_____

_____

Two Hour Glucose Reading:_____

Mid Afternoon Snack:_____

Dinner:

Time:_____Total Carbs:_____

_____

_____

_____

Two Hour Glucose Reading:_____

Evening Snack:_____

Date:_____

A.M. Glucose Reading:_____

Breakfast:

Time:_____ Total Carbs:_____
_____
_____
_____

Two Hour Glucose Reading:_____
Mid Morning Snack:_____

Lunch:

Time:_____ Total Carbs:_____
_____
_____
_____

Two Hour Glucose Reading:_____
Mid Afternoon Snack:_____

Dinner:

Time:_____Total Carbs:_____
_____
_____
_____

Two Hour Glucose Reading:_____
Evening Snack:_____

Date:_____

A.M. Glucose Reading:_____

Breakfast:

Time:_____     Total Carbs:_____
_____
_____
_____

Two Hour Glucose Reading:_____
Mid Morning Snack:_____

Lunch:

Time:_____     Total Carbs:_____
_____
_____
_____

Two Hour Glucose Reading:_____
Mid Afternoon Snack:_____

Dinner:

Time:_____Total Carbs:_____
_____
_____
_____

Two Hour Glucose Reading:_____
Evening Snack:_____

Date:_____

A.M. Glucose Reading:_____

Breakfast:

Time:_____ Total Carbs:_____

_____
_____
_____

Two Hour Glucose Reading:_____
Mid Morning Snack:_____

Lunch:

Time:_____ Total Carbs:_____

_____
_____
_____

Two Hour Glucose Reading:_____
Mid Afternoon Snack:_____

Dinner:

Time:_____Total Carbs:_____

_____
_____
_____

Two Hour Glucose Reading:_____
Evening Snack:_____

Date:_____

A.M. Glucose Reading:_____

---

Breakfast:

Time:_____ Total Carbs:_____

_____

_____

_____

Two Hour Glucose Reading:_____

Mid Morning Snack:_____

---

Lunch:

Time:_____ Total Carbs:_____

_____

_____

_____

Two Hour Glucose Reading:_____

Mid Afternoon Snack:_____

---

Dinner:

Time:_____Total Carbs:_____

_____

_____

_____

Two Hour Glucose Reading:_____

Evening Snack:_____

Date:_____

A.M. Glucose Reading:_____

Breakfast:

Time:_____ Total Carbs:_____

_____
_____
_____

Two Hour Glucose Reading:_____
Mid Morning Snack:_____

Lunch:

Time:_____ Total Carbs:_____

_____
_____
_____

Two Hour Glucose Reading:_____
Mid Afternoon Snack:_____

Dinner:

Time:_____Total Carbs:_____

_____
_____
_____

Two Hour Glucose Reading:_____
Evening Snack:_____

Date:_____

A.M. Glucose Reading:_____

Breakfast:

Time:_____ Total Carbs:_____

_____
_____
_____

Two Hour Glucose Reading:_____
Mid Morning Snack:_____

Lunch:

Time:_____ Total Carbs:_____

_____
_____
_____

Two Hour Glucose Reading:_____
Mid Afternoon Snack:_____

Dinner:

Time:_____Total Carbs:_____

_____
_____
_____

Two Hour Glucose Reading:_____
Evening Snack:_____

Date:_____

A.M. Glucose Reading:_____

Breakfast:

Time:_____ Total Carbs:_____

_____
_____
_____

Two Hour Glucose Reading:_____
Mid Morning Snack:_____

Lunch:

Time:_____ Total Carbs:_____

_____
_____
_____

Two Hour Glucose Reading:_____
Mid Afternoon Snack:_____

Dinner:

Time:_____Total Carbs:_____

_____
_____
_____

Two Hour Glucose Reading:_____
Evening Snack:_____

Date:_____

A.M. Glucose Reading:_____

Breakfast:

Time:_____ Total Carbs:_____

_____

_____

_____

Two Hour Glucose Reading:_____

Mid Morning Snack:_____

Lunch:

Time:_____ Total Carbs:_____

_____

_____

_____

Two Hour Glucose Reading:_____

Mid Afternoon Snack:_____

Dinner:

Time:_____Total Carbs:_____

_____

_____

_____

Two Hour Glucose Reading:_____

Evening Snack:_____

Date:_____

A.M. Glucose Reading:_____

Breakfast:

Time:_____ Total Carbs:_____
_____
_____
_____

Two Hour Glucose Reading:_____
Mid Morning Snack:_____

Lunch:

Time:_____ Total Carbs:_____
_____
_____
_____

Two Hour Glucose Reading:_____
Mid Afternoon Snack:_____

Dinner:

Time:_____Total Carbs:_____
_____
_____
_____

Two Hour Glucose Reading:_____
Evening Snack:_____

Date:_____

A.M. Glucose Reading:_____

Breakfast:

Time:_____ Total Carbs:_____
_____
_____
_____
Two Hour Glucose Reading:_____
Mid Morning Snack:_____

Lunch:

Time:_____ Total Carbs:_____
_____
_____
_____
Two Hour Glucose Reading:_____
Mid Afternoon Snack:_____

Dinner:

Time:_____Total Carbs:_____
_____
_____
_____
Two Hour Glucose Reading:_____
Evening Snack:_____

Date:_____

A.M. Glucose Reading:_____

Breakfast:

Time:_____  Total Carbs:_____

_____
_____
_____

Two Hour Glucose Reading:_____
Mid Morning Snack:_____

Lunch:

Time:_____  Total Carbs:_____

_____
_____
_____

Two Hour Glucose Reading:_____
Mid Afternoon Snack:_____

Dinner:

Time:_____Total Carbs:_____

_____
_____
_____

Two Hour Glucose Reading:_____
Evening Snack:_____

Date:_____

A.M. Glucose Reading:_____

Breakfast:

Time:_____ Total Carbs:_____
_____
_____
_____

Two Hour Glucose Reading:_____
Mid Morning Snack:_____

Lunch:

Time:_____ Total Carbs:_____
_____
_____
_____

Two Hour Glucose Reading:_____
Mid Afternoon Snack:_____

Dinner:

Time:_____Total Carbs:_____
_____
_____
_____

Two Hour Glucose Reading:_____
Evening Snack:_____

Date:_____

A.M. Glucose Reading:_____

Breakfast:

Time:_____ Total Carbs:_____

_____

_____

_____

Two Hour Glucose Reading:_____

Mid Morning Snack:_____

Lunch:

Time:_____ Total Carbs:_____

_____

_____

_____

Two Hour Glucose Reading:_____

Mid Afternoon Snack:_____

Dinner:

Time:_____Total Carbs:_____

_____

_____

_____

Two Hour Glucose Reading:_____

Evening Snack:_____

Date:_____

A.M. Glucose Reading:_____

Breakfast:

Time:_____ Total Carbs:_____
_____
_____
_____

Two Hour Glucose Reading:_____
Mid Morning Snack:_____

Lunch:

Time:_____ Total Carbs:_____
_____
_____
_____

Two Hour Glucose Reading:_____
Mid Afternoon Snack:_____

Dinner:

Time:_____Total Carbs:_____
_____
_____
_____

Two Hour Glucose Reading:_____
Evening Snack:_____

Date:_____

A.M. Glucose Reading:_____

---

Breakfast:

Time:_____ Total Carbs:_____

_____
_____
_____

Two Hour Glucose Reading:_____
Mid Morning Snack:_____

---

Lunch:

Time:_____ Total Carbs:_____

_____
_____
_____

Two Hour Glucose Reading:_____
Mid Afternoon Snack:_____

---

Dinner:

Time:_____Total Carbs:_____

_____
_____
_____

Two Hour Glucose Reading:_____
Evening Snack:_____

Date:_____

A.M. Glucose Reading:_____

---

Breakfast:

Time:_____ Total Carbs:_____

_____

_____

_____

Two Hour Glucose Reading:_____

Mid Morning Snack:_____

---

Lunch:

Time:_____ Total Carbs:_____

_____

_____

_____

Two Hour Glucose Reading:_____

Mid Afternoon Snack:_____

---

Dinner:

Time:_____Total Carbs:_____

_____

_____

_____

Two Hour Glucose Reading:_____

Evening Snack:_____

Date:_____

A.M. Glucose Reading:_____

Breakfast:

Time:_____    Total Carbs:_____

_____
_____
_____

Two Hour Glucose Reading:_____
Mid Morning Snack:_____

Lunch:

Time:_____    Total Carbs:_____

_____
_____
_____

Two Hour Glucose Reading:_____
Mid Afternoon Snack:_____

Dinner:

Time:_____Total Carbs:_____

_____
_____
_____

Two Hour Glucose Reading:_____
Evening Snack:_____

Date:_____

A.M. Glucose Reading:_____

Breakfast:

Time:_____ Total Carbs:_____
_____
_____
_____

Two Hour Glucose Reading:_____
Mid Morning Snack:_____

Lunch:

Time:_____ Total Carbs:_____
_____
_____
_____

Two Hour Glucose Reading:_____
Mid Afternoon Snack:_____

Dinner:

Time:_____Total Carbs:_____
_____
_____
_____

Two Hour Glucose Reading:_____
Evening Snack:_____

Date:_____

A.M. Glucose Reading:_____

Breakfast:

Time:_____ Total Carbs:_____

_____

_____

_____

Two Hour Glucose Reading:_____
Mid Morning Snack:_____

Lunch:

Time:_____ Total Carbs:_____

_____

_____

_____

Two Hour Glucose Reading:_____
Mid Afternoon Snack:_____

Dinner:

Time:_____Total Carbs:_____

_____

_____

_____

Two Hour Glucose Reading:_____
Evening Snack:_____

Date:_____

A.M. Glucose Reading:_____

Breakfast:

Time:_____ Total Carbs:_____

_____
_____
_____

Two Hour Glucose Reading:_____

Mid Morning Snack:_____

Lunch:

Time:_____ Total Carbs:_____

_____
_____
_____

Two Hour Glucose Reading:_____

Mid Afternoon Snack:_____

Dinner:

Time:_____Total Carbs:_____

_____
_____
_____

Two Hour Glucose Reading:_____

Evening Snack:_____

Date:_____

A.M. Glucose Reading:_____

Breakfast:

Time:_____ Total Carbs:_____
_____
_____
_____

Two Hour Glucose Reading:_____
Mid Morning Snack:_____

Lunch:

Time:_____ Total Carbs:_____
_____
_____
_____

Two Hour Glucose Reading:_____
Mid Afternoon Snack:_____

Dinner:

Time:_____Total Carbs:_____
_____
_____
_____

Two Hour Glucose Reading:_____
Evening Snack:_____

Date:_____

A.M. Glucose Reading:_____

Breakfast:

Time:_____ Total Carbs:_____

_____

_____

_____

Two Hour Glucose Reading:_____

Mid Morning Snack:_____

Lunch:

Time:_____ Total Carbs:_____

_____

_____

_____

Two Hour Glucose Reading:_____

Mid Afternoon Snack:_____

Dinner:

Time:_____Total Carbs:_____

_____

_____

_____

Two Hour Glucose Reading:_____

Evening Snack:_____

Date:_____

A.M. Glucose Reading:_____

Breakfast:

Time:_____ Total Carbs:_____

_____
_____
_____

Two Hour Glucose Reading:_____
Mid Morning Snack:_____

Lunch:

Time:_____ Total Carbs:_____

_____
_____
_____

Two Hour Glucose Reading:_____
Mid Afternoon Snack:_____

Dinner:

Time:_____ Total Carbs:_____

_____
_____
_____

Two Hour Glucose Reading:_____
Evening Snack:_____

Date:_____

A.M. Glucose Reading:_____

Breakfast:

Time:_____  Total Carbs:_____

_____

_____

_____

Two Hour Glucose Reading:_____

Mid Morning Snack:_____

Lunch:

Time:_____  Total Carbs:_____

_____

_____

_____

Two Hour Glucose Reading:_____

Mid Afternoon Snack:_____

Dinner:

Time:_____Total Carbs:_____

_____

_____

_____

Two Hour Glucose Reading:_____

Evening Snack:_____

Date:_____

A.M. Glucose Reading:_____

Breakfast:

Time:_____ Total Carbs:_____

_____
_____
_____

Two Hour Glucose Reading:_____
Mid Morning Snack:_____

Lunch:

Time:_____ Total Carbs:_____

_____
_____
_____

Two Hour Glucose Reading:_____
Mid Afternoon Snack:_____

Dinner:

Time:_____Total Carbs:_____

_____
_____
_____

Two Hour Glucose Reading:_____
Evening Snack:_____

Date:_____

A.M. Glucose Reading:_____

Breakfast:

Time:_____ Total Carbs:_____
_____
_____
_____
Two Hour Glucose Reading:_____
Mid Morning Snack:_____

Lunch:

Time:_____ Total Carbs:_____
_____
_____
_____
Two Hour Glucose Reading:_____
Mid Afternoon Snack:_____

Dinner:

Time:_____Total Carbs:_____
_____
_____
_____
Two Hour Glucose Reading:_____
Evening Snack:_____

Date:_____

A.M. Glucose Reading:_____

Breakfast:

Time:_____    Total Carbs:_____

_____
_____
_____

Two Hour Glucose Reading:_____
Mid Morning Snack:_____

Lunch:

Time:_____    Total Carbs:_____

_____
_____
_____

Two Hour Glucose Reading:_____
Mid Afternoon Snack:_____

Dinner:

Time:_____Total Carbs:_____

_____
_____
_____

Two Hour Glucose Reading:_____
Evening Snack:_____

Date:_____

A.M. Glucose Reading:_____

Breakfast:

Time:_____ Total Carbs:_____

_____
_____
_____

Two Hour Glucose Reading:_____
Mid Morning Snack:_____

Lunch:

Time:_____ Total Carbs:_____

_____
_____
_____

Two Hour Glucose Reading:_____
Mid Afternoon Snack:_____

Dinner:

Time:_____Total Carbs:_____

_____
_____
_____

Two Hour Glucose Reading:_____
Evening Snack:_____

Date:_____

A.M. Glucose Reading:_____

Breakfast:

Time:_____ Total Carbs:_____

_____

_____

_____

Two Hour Glucose Reading:_____

Mid Morning Snack:_____

Lunch:

Time:_____ Total Carbs:_____

_____

_____

_____

Two Hour Glucose Reading:_____

Mid Afternoon Snack:_____

Dinner:

Time:_____Total Carbs:_____

_____

_____

_____

Two Hour Glucose Reading:_____

Evening Snack:_____

Date:_____

A.M. Glucose Reading:_____

Breakfast:

Time:_____ Total Carbs:_____

_____
_____
_____

Two Hour Glucose Reading:_____
Mid Morning Snack:_____

Lunch:

Time:_____ Total Carbs:_____

_____
_____
_____

Two Hour Glucose Reading:_____
Mid Afternoon Snack:_____

Dinner:

Time:_____Total Carbs:_____

_____
_____
_____

Two Hour Glucose Reading:_____
Evening Snack:_____

Date:_____

A.M. Glucose Reading:_____

---

Breakfast:

Time:_____    Total Carbs:_____

_____
_____
_____

Two Hour Glucose Reading:_____
Mid Morning Snack:_____

---

Lunch:

Time:_____    Total Carbs:_____

_____
_____
_____

Two Hour Glucose Reading:_____
Mid Afternoon Snack:_____

---

Dinner:

Time:_____Total Carbs:_____

_____
_____
_____

Two Hour Glucose Reading:_____
Evening Snack:_____

Date:_____

A.M. Glucose Reading:_____

Breakfast:

Time:_____ Total Carbs:_____
_____
_____
_____

Two Hour Glucose Reading:_____
Mid Morning Snack:_____

Lunch:

Time:_____ Total Carbs:_____
_____
_____
_____

Two Hour Glucose Reading:_____
Mid Afternoon Snack:_____

Dinner:

Time:_____Total Carbs:_____
_____
_____
_____

Two Hour Glucose Reading:_____
Evening Snack:_____

Date:_____

A.M. Glucose Reading:_____

Breakfast:

Time:_____ Total Carbs:_____

_____

_____

_____

Two Hour Glucose Reading:_____

Mid Morning Snack:_____

Lunch:

Time:_____ Total Carbs:_____

_____

_____

_____

Two Hour Glucose Reading:_____

Mid Afternoon Snack:_____

Dinner:

Time:_____Total Carbs:_____

_____

_____

_____

Two Hour Glucose Reading:_____

Evening Snack:_____

Date:_____

A.M. Glucose Reading:_____

Breakfast:

Time:_____  Total Carbs:_____

_____

_____

_____

Two Hour Glucose Reading:_____

Mid Morning Snack:_____

Lunch:

Time:_____  Total Carbs:_____

_____

_____

_____

Two Hour Glucose Reading:_____
Mid Afternoon Snack:_____

Dinner:

Time:_____  Total Carbs:_____

_____

_____

_____

Two Hour Glucose Reading:_____
Evening Snack:_____

Date:_____

A.M. Glucose Reading:_____

Breakfast:

Time:_____ Total Carbs:_____

_____
_____
_____

Two Hour Glucose Reading:_____
Mid Morning Snack:_____

Lunch:

Time:_____ Total Carbs:_____

_____
_____
_____

Two Hour Glucose Reading:_____
Mid Afternoon Snack:_____

Dinner:

Time:_____Total Carbs:_____

_____
_____
_____

Two Hour Glucose Reading:_____
Evening Snack:_____

Date:_____

A.M. Glucose Reading:_____

Breakfast:

Time:_____ Total Carbs:_____
_____
_____
_____

Two Hour Glucose Reading:_____
Mid Morning Snack:_____

Lunch:

Time:_____ Total Carbs:_____
_____
_____
_____

Two Hour Glucose Reading:_____
Mid Afternoon Snack:_____

Dinner:

Time:_____Total Carbs:_____
_____
_____
_____

Two Hour Glucose Reading:_____
Evening Snack:_____

Date:_____

A.M. Glucose Reading:_____

Breakfast:

Time:_____ Total Carbs:_____
_____
_____
_____

Two Hour Glucose Reading:_____
Mid Morning Snack:_____

Lunch:

Time:_____ Total Carbs:_____
_____
_____
_____

Two Hour Glucose Reading:_____
Mid Afternoon Snack:_____

Dinner:

Time:_____Total Carbs:_____
_____
_____
_____

Two Hour Glucose Reading:_____
Evening Snack:_____

Date:_____

A.M. Glucose Reading:_____

---

Breakfast:

Time:_____     Total Carbs:_____

_____

_____

_____

Two Hour Glucose Reading:_____

Mid Morning Snack:_____

---

Lunch:

Time:_____     Total Carbs:_____

_____

_____

_____

Two Hour Glucose Reading:_____

Mid Afternoon Snack:_____

---

Dinner:

Time:_____Total Carbs:_____

_____

_____

_____

Two Hour Glucose Reading:_____

Evening Snack:_____

Date:_____

A.M. Glucose Reading:_____

Breakfast:

Time:_____ Total Carbs:_____
_____
_____
_____

Two Hour Glucose Reading:_____
Mid Morning Snack:_____

Lunch:

Time:_____ Total Carbs:_____
_____
_____
_____

Two Hour Glucose Reading:_____
Mid Afternoon Snack:_____

Dinner:

Time:_____Total Carbs:_____
_____
_____
_____

Two Hour Glucose Reading:_____
Evening Snack:_____

Date:_____

A.M. Glucose Reading:_____

Breakfast:

Time:_____ Total Carbs:_____
_____
_____
_____

Two Hour Glucose Reading:_____
Mid Morning Snack:_____

Lunch:

Time:_____ Total Carbs:_____
_____
_____
_____

Two Hour Glucose Reading:_____
Mid Afternoon Snack:_____

Dinner:

Time:_____Total Carbs:_____
_____
_____
_____

Two Hour Glucose Reading:_____
Evening Snack:_____

Date:_____

A.M. Glucose Reading:_____

Breakfast:

Time:_____  Total Carbs:_____

_____
_____
_____

Two Hour Glucose Reading:_____
Mid Morning Snack:_____

Lunch:

Time:_____  Total Carbs:_____

_____
_____
_____

Two Hour Glucose Reading:_____
Mid Afternoon Snack:_____

Dinner:

Time:_____Total Carbs:_____

_____
_____
_____

Two Hour Glucose Reading:_____
Evening Snack:_____

Date:_____

A.M. Glucose Reading:_____

---

Breakfast:

Time:_____ Total Carbs:_____

_____

_____

_____

Two Hour Glucose Reading:_____

Mid Morning Snack:_____

---

Lunch:

Time:_____ Total Carbs:_____

_____

_____

_____

Two Hour Glucose Reading:_____

Mid Afternoon Snack:_____

---

Dinner:

Time:_____Total Carbs:_____

_____

_____

_____

Two Hour Glucose Reading:_____

Evening Snack:_____

Date:_____

A.M. Glucose Reading:_____

Breakfast:

Time:_____ Total Carbs:_____
_____
_____
_____

Two Hour Glucose Reading:_____
Mid Morning Snack:_____

Lunch:

Time:_____ Total Carbs:_____
_____
_____
_____

Two Hour Glucose Reading:_____
Mid Afternoon Snack:_____

Dinner:

Time:_____Total Carbs:_____
_____
_____
_____

Two Hour Glucose Reading:_____
Evening Snack:_____

Date:_____

A.M. Glucose Reading:_____

Breakfast:

Time:_____ Total Carbs:_____

_____
_____
_____

Two Hour Glucose Reading:_____
Mid Morning Snack:_____

Lunch:

Time:_____ Total Carbs:_____

_____
_____
_____

Two Hour Glucose Reading:_____
Mid Afternoon Snack:_____

Dinner:

Time:_____Total Carbs:_____

_____
_____
_____

Two Hour Glucose Reading:_____
Evening Snack:_____

Date:_____

A.M. Glucose Reading:_____

Breakfast:

Time:_____ Total Carbs:_____

_____
_____
_____

Two Hour Glucose Reading:_____
Mid Morning Snack:_____

Lunch:

Time:_____ Total Carbs:_____

_____
_____
_____

Two Hour Glucose Reading:_____
Mid Afternoon Snack:_____

Dinner:

Time:_____Total Carbs:_____

_____
_____
_____

Two Hour Glucose Reading:_____
Evening Snack:_____

Date:_____

A.M. Glucose Reading:_____

Breakfast:

Time:_____ Total Carbs:_____

_____

_____

_____

Two Hour Glucose Reading:_____

Mid Morning Snack:_____

---

Lunch:

Time:_____ Total Carbs:_____

_____

_____

_____

Two Hour Glucose Reading:_____

Mid Afternoon Snack:_____

---

Dinner:

Time:_____Total Carbs:_____

_____

_____

_____

Two Hour Glucose Reading:_____

Evening Snack:_____

Date:_____

A.M. Glucose Reading:_____

Breakfast:

Time:_____     Total Carbs:_____
_____
_____
_____

Two Hour Glucose Reading:_____
Mid Morning Snack:_____

Lunch:

Time:_____     Total Carbs:_____
_____
_____
_____

Two Hour Glucose Reading:_____
Mid Afternoon Snack:_____

Dinner:

Time:_____Total Carbs:_____
_____
_____
_____

Two Hour Glucose Reading:_____
Evening Snack:_____

Date:_____

A.M. Glucose Reading:_____

Breakfast:

Time:_____ Total Carbs:_____

_____

_____

_____

Two Hour Glucose Reading:_____

Mid Morning Snack:_____

Lunch:

Time:_____ Total Carbs:_____

_____

_____

_____

Two Hour Glucose Reading:_____

Mid Afternoon Snack:_____

Dinner:

Time:_____Total Carbs:_____

_____

_____

_____

Two Hour Glucose Reading:_____

Evening Snack:_____

Date:_____

A.M. Glucose Reading:_____

Breakfast:

Time:_____ Total Carbs:_____
_____
_____
_____

Two Hour Glucose Reading:_____
Mid Morning Snack:_____

Lunch:

Time:_____ Total Carbs:_____
_____
_____
_____

Two Hour Glucose Reading:_____
Mid Afternoon Snack:_____

Dinner:

Time:_____Total Carbs:_____
_____
_____
_____

Two Hour Glucose Reading:_____
Evening Snack:_____

Date:_____

A.M. Glucose Reading:_____

---

Breakfast:

Time:_____     Total Carbs:_____

_____

_____

_____

Two Hour Glucose Reading:_____

Mid Morning Snack:_____

---

Lunch:

Time:_____     Total Carbs:_____

_____

_____

_____

Two Hour Glucose Reading:_____

Mid Afternoon Snack:_____

---

Dinner:

Time:_____Total Carbs:_____

_____

_____

_____

Two Hour Glucose Reading:_____

Evening Snack:_____

Date:_____

A.M. Glucose Reading:_____

Breakfast:

Time:_____ Total Carbs:_____

_____

_____

_____

Two Hour Glucose Reading:_____

Mid Morning Snack:_____

Lunch:

Time:_____ Total Carbs:_____

_____

_____

_____

Two Hour Glucose Reading:_____

Mid Afternoon Snack:_____

Dinner:

Time:_____Total Carbs:_____

_____

_____

_____

Two Hour Glucose Reading:_____

Evening Snack:_____

Date:_____

A.M. Glucose Reading:_____

Breakfast:

Time:_____ Total Carbs:_____

_____
_____
_____

Two Hour Glucose Reading:_____
Mid Morning Snack:_____

Lunch:

Time:_____ Total Carbs:_____

_____
_____
_____

Two Hour Glucose Reading:_____
Mid Afternoon Snack:_____

Dinner:

Time:_____Total Carbs:_____

_____
_____
_____

Two Hour Glucose Reading:_____
Evening Snack:_____

Date:_____

A.M. Glucose Reading:_____

Breakfast:

Time:_____ Total Carbs:_____
_____
_____
_____

Two Hour Glucose Reading:_____
Mid Morning Snack:_____

Lunch:

Time:_____ Total Carbs:_____
_____
_____
_____

Two Hour Glucose Reading:_____
Mid Afternoon Snack:_____

Dinner:

Time:_____Total Carbs:_____
_____
_____
_____

Two Hour Glucose Reading:_____
Evening Snack:_____

Date:_____

A.M. Glucose Reading:_____

Breakfast:

Time:_____ Total Carbs:_____

_____
_____
_____

Two Hour Glucose Reading:_____
Mid Morning Snack:_____

Lunch:

Time:_____ Total Carbs:_____

_____
_____
_____

Two Hour Glucose Reading:_____
Mid Afternoon Snack:_____

Dinner:

Time:_____Total Carbs:_____

_____
_____
_____

Two Hour Glucose Reading:_____
Evening Snack:_____

Date:_____

A.M. Glucose Reading:_____

Breakfast:

Time:_____ Total Carbs:_____
_____
_____
_____

Two Hour Glucose Reading:_____
Mid Morning Snack:_____

Lunch:

Time:_____ Total Carbs:_____
_____
_____
_____

Two Hour Glucose Reading:_____
Mid Afternoon Snack:_____

Dinner:

Time:_____Total Carbs:_____
_____
_____
_____

Two Hour Glucose Reading:_____
Evening Snack:_____

Date:_____

A.M. Glucose Reading:_____

Breakfast:

Time:_____ Total Carbs:_____

_____
_____
_____

Two Hour Glucose Reading:_____
Mid Morning Snack:_____

Lunch:

Time:_____ Total Carbs:_____

_____
_____
_____

Two Hour Glucose Reading:_____
Mid Afternoon Snack:_____

Dinner:

Time:_____ Total Carbs:_____

_____
_____
_____

Two Hour Glucose Reading:_____
Evening Snack:_____

Date:_____

A.M. Glucose Reading:_____

---

Breakfast:

Time:_____  Total Carbs:_____

_____

_____

_____

Two Hour Glucose Reading:_____

Mid Morning Snack:_____

---

Lunch:

Time:_____  Total Carbs:_____

_____

_____

_____

Two Hour Glucose Reading:_____

Mid Afternoon Snack:_____

---

Dinner:

Time:_____  Total Carbs:_____

_____

_____

_____

Two Hour Glucose Reading:_____

Evening Snack:_____

Date:_____

A.M. Glucose Reading:_____

Breakfast:

Time:_____ Total Carbs:_____

_____
_____
_____

Two Hour Glucose Reading:_____
Mid Morning Snack:_____

Lunch:

Time:_____ Total Carbs:_____

_____
_____
_____

Two Hour Glucose Reading:_____
Mid Afternoon Snack:_____

Dinner:

Time:_____Total Carbs:_____

_____
_____
_____

Two Hour Glucose Reading:_____
Evening Snack:_____

Date:_____

A.M. Glucose Reading:_____

Breakfast:

Time:_____ Total Carbs:_____
_____
_____
_____

Two Hour Glucose Reading:_____
Mid Morning Snack:_____

Lunch:

Time:_____ Total Carbs:_____
_____
_____
_____

Two Hour Glucose Reading:_____
Mid Afternoon Snack:_____

Dinner:

Time:_____Total Carbs:_____
_____
_____
_____

Two Hour Glucose Reading:_____
Evening Snack:_____

Date:_____

A.M. Glucose Reading:_____

Breakfast:

Time:_____ Total Carbs:_____

_____
_____
_____

Two Hour Glucose Reading:_____
Mid Morning Snack:_____

Lunch:

Time:_____ Total Carbs:_____

_____
_____
_____

Two Hour Glucose Reading:_____
Mid Afternoon Snack:_____

Dinner:

Time:_____Total Carbs:_____

_____
_____
_____

Two Hour Glucose Reading:_____
Evening Snack:_____

Date:_____

A.M. Glucose Reading:_____

---

Breakfast:

Time:_____  Total Carbs:_____

_____
_____
_____

Two Hour Glucose Reading:_____
Mid Morning Snack:_____

---

Lunch:

Time:_____  Total Carbs:_____

_____
_____
_____

Two Hour Glucose Reading:_____
Mid Afternoon Snack:_____

---

Dinner:

Time:_____Total Carbs:_____

_____
_____
_____

Two Hour Glucose Reading:_____
Evening Snack:_____

Date:_____

A.M. Glucose Reading:_____

---

**Breakfast:**

Time:_____  Total Carbs:_____

_____

_____

_____

Two Hour Glucose Reading:_____

Mid Morning Snack:_____

---

**Lunch:**

Time:_____  Total Carbs:_____

_____

_____

_____

Two Hour Glucose Reading:_____

Mid Afternoon Snack:_____

---

**Dinner:**

Time:_____Total Carbs:_____

_____

_____

_____

Two Hour Glucose Reading:_____

Evening Snack:_____

Date:_____

A.M. Glucose Reading:_____

Breakfast:

Time:_____ Total Carbs:_____

_____

_____

_____

Two Hour Glucose Reading:_____
Mid Morning Snack:_____

Lunch:

Time:_____ Total Carbs:_____

_____

_____

_____

Two Hour Glucose Reading:_____
Mid Afternoon Snack:_____

Dinner:

Time:_____Total Carbs:_____

_____

_____

_____

Two Hour Glucose Reading:_____
Evening Snack:_____

Date:_____

A.M. Glucose Reading:_____

Breakfast:

Time:_____ Total Carbs:_____

_____

_____

_____

Two Hour Glucose Reading:_____

Mid Morning Snack:_____

Lunch:

Time:_____ Total Carbs:_____

_____

_____

_____

Two Hour Glucose Reading:_____

Mid Afternoon Snack:_____

Dinner:

Time:_____ Total Carbs:_____

_____

_____

_____

Two Hour Glucose Reading:_____

Evening Snack:_____

Date:_____

A.M. Glucose Reading:_____

Breakfast:

Time:_____    Total Carbs:_____
_____
_____
_____

Two Hour Glucose Reading:_____
Mid Morning Snack:_____

Lunch:

Time:_____    Total Carbs:_____
_____
_____
_____

Two Hour Glucose Reading:_____
Mid Afternoon Snack:_____

Dinner:

Time:_____Total Carbs:_____
_____
_____
_____

Two Hour Glucose Reading:_____
Evening Snack:_____

Date:_____

A.M. Glucose Reading:_____

---

Breakfast:

Time:_____     Total Carbs:_____
_____
_____
_____

Two Hour Glucose Reading:_____
Mid Morning Snack:_____

---

Lunch:

Time:_____     Total Carbs:_____
_____
_____
_____

Two Hour Glucose Reading:_____
Mid Afternoon Snack:_____

---

Dinner:

Time:_____     Total Carbs:_____
_____
_____
_____

Two Hour Glucose Reading:_____
Evening Snack:_____

Date:_____

A.M. Glucose Reading:_____

Breakfast:

Time:_____ Total Carbs:_____
_____
_____
_____

Two Hour Glucose Reading:_____
Mid Morning Snack:_____

Lunch:

Time:_____ Total Carbs:_____
_____
_____
_____

Two Hour Glucose Reading:_____
Mid Afternoon Snack:_____

Dinner:

Time:_____Total Carbs:_____
_____
_____
_____

Two Hour Glucose Reading:_____
Evening Snack:_____

Date:_____

A.M. Glucose Reading:_____

Breakfast:

Time:_____  Total Carbs:_____

_____

_____

_____

Two Hour Glucose Reading:_____

Mid Morning Snack:_____

Lunch:

Time:_____  Total Carbs:_____

_____

_____

_____

Two Hour Glucose Reading:_____

Mid Afternoon Snack:_____

Dinner:

Time:_____Total Carbs:_____

_____

_____

_____

Two Hour Glucose Reading:_____

Evening Snack:_____

Date:_____

A.M. Glucose Reading:_____

Breakfast:

Time:_____ Total Carbs:_____

_____

_____

_____

Two Hour Glucose Reading:_____
Mid Morning Snack:_____

Lunch:

Time:_____ Total Carbs:_____

_____

_____

_____

Two Hour Glucose Reading:_____
Mid Afternoon Snack:_____

Dinner:

Time:_____Total Carbs:_____

_____

_____

_____

Two Hour Glucose Reading:_____
Evening Snack:_____

Date:_____

A.M. Glucose Reading:_____

---

Breakfast:

Time:_____ Total Carbs:_____

_____
_____
_____

Two Hour Glucose Reading:_____
Mid Morning Snack:_____

---

Lunch:

Time:_____ Total Carbs:_____

_____
_____
_____

Two Hour Glucose Reading:_____
Mid Afternoon Snack:_____

---

Dinner:

Time:_____ Total Carbs:_____

_____
_____
_____

Two Hour Glucose Reading:_____
Evening Snack:_____

Date:_____

A.M. Glucose Reading:_____

Breakfast:

Time:_____  Total Carbs:_____
_____
_____
_____

Two Hour Glucose Reading:_____
Mid Morning Snack:_____

Lunch:

Time:_____  Total Carbs:_____
_____
_____
_____

Two Hour Glucose Reading:_____
Mid Afternoon Snack:_____

Dinner:

Time:_____  Total Carbs:_____
_____
_____
_____

Two Hour Glucose Reading:_____
Evening Snack:_____

Date:_____

A.M. Glucose Reading:_____

Breakfast:

Time:_____ Total Carbs:_____

_____
_____
_____

Two Hour Glucose Reading:_____
Mid Morning Snack:_____

Lunch:

Time:_____ Total Carbs:_____

_____
_____
_____

Two Hour Glucose Reading:_____
Mid Afternoon Snack:_____

Dinner:

Time:_____Total Carbs:_____

_____
_____
_____

Two Hour Glucose Reading:_____
Evening Snack:_____

Date:_____

A.M. Glucose Reading:_____

Breakfast:

Time:_____ Total Carbs:_____

_____

_____

_____

Two Hour Glucose Reading:_____

Mid Morning Snack:_____

Lunch:

Time:_____ Total Carbs:_____

_____

_____

_____

Two Hour Glucose Reading:_____

Mid Afternoon Snack:_____

Dinner:

Time:_____Total Carbs:_____

_____

_____

_____

Two Hour Glucose Reading:_____

Evening Snack:_____

Date:_____

A.M. Glucose Reading:_____

---

Breakfast:

Time:_____  Total Carbs:_____

_____
_____
_____

Two Hour Glucose Reading:_____

Mid Morning Snack:_____

---

Lunch:

Time:_____  Total Carbs:_____

_____
_____
_____

Two Hour Glucose Reading:_____

Mid Afternoon Snack:_____

---

Dinner:

Time:_____Total Carbs:_____

_____
_____
_____

Two Hour Glucose Reading:_____

Evening Snack:_____

Date:_____

A.M. Glucose Reading:_____

Breakfast:

Time:_____ Total Carbs:_____
_____
_____
_____

Two Hour Glucose Reading:_____
Mid Morning Snack:_____

Lunch:

Time:_____ Total Carbs:_____
_____
_____
_____

Two Hour Glucose Reading:_____
Mid Afternoon Snack:_____

Dinner:

Time:_____Total Carbs:_____
_____
_____
_____

Two Hour Glucose Reading:_____
Evening Snack:_____

Date:_____

A.M. Glucose Reading:_____

Breakfast:

Time:_____ Total Carbs:_____
_____
_____
_____

Two Hour Glucose Reading:_____
Mid Morning Snack:_____

Lunch:

Time:_____ Total Carbs:_____
_____
_____
_____

Two Hour Glucose Reading:_____
Mid Afternoon Snack:_____

Dinner:

Time:_____Total Carbs:_____
_____
_____
_____

Two Hour Glucose Reading:_____
Evening Snack:_____

Date:_____

A.M. Glucose Reading:_____

Breakfast:

Time:_____ Total Carbs:_____

_____

_____

_____

Two Hour Glucose Reading:_____

Mid Morning Snack:_____

Lunch:

Time:_____ Total Carbs:_____

_____

_____

_____

Two Hour Glucose Reading:_____

Mid Afternoon Snack:_____

Dinner:

Time:_____Total Carbs:_____

_____

_____

_____

Two Hour Glucose Reading:_____

Evening Snack:_____

Date:_____

A.M. Glucose Reading:_____

Breakfast:

Time:_____ Total Carbs:_____

_____
_____
_____

Two Hour Glucose Reading:_____
Mid Morning Snack:_____

Lunch:

Time:_____ Total Carbs:_____

_____
_____
_____

Two Hour Glucose Reading:_____
Mid Afternoon Snack:_____

Dinner:

Time:_____Total Carbs:_____

_____
_____
_____

Two Hour Glucose Reading:_____
Evening Snack:_____

Date:_____

A.M. Glucose Reading:_____

Breakfast:

Time:_____ Total Carbs:_____
_____
_____
_____

Two Hour Glucose Reading:_____
Mid Morning Snack:_____

Lunch:

Time:_____ Total Carbs:_____
_____
_____
_____

Two Hour Glucose Reading:_____
Mid Afternoon Snack:_____

Dinner:

Time:_____Total Carbs:_____
_____
_____
_____

Two Hour Glucose Reading:_____
Evening Snack:_____

Date:_____

A.M. Glucose Reading:_____

Breakfast:

Time:_____  Total Carbs:_____

_____
_____
_____

Two Hour Glucose Reading:_____
Mid Morning Snack:_____

Lunch:

Time:_____  Total Carbs:_____

_____
_____
_____

Two Hour Glucose Reading:_____
Mid Afternoon Snack:_____

Dinner:

Time:_____Total Carbs:_____

_____
_____
_____

Two Hour Glucose Reading:_____
Evening Snack:_____

Date:_____

A.M. Glucose Reading:_____

Breakfast:

Time:_____ Total Carbs:_____
_____
_____
_____

Two Hour Glucose Reading:_____
Mid Morning Snack:_____

Lunch:

Time:_____ Total Carbs:_____
_____
_____
_____

Two Hour Glucose Reading:_____
Mid Afternoon Snack:_____

Dinner:

Time:_____Total Carbs:_____
_____
_____
_____

Two Hour Glucose Reading:_____
Evening Snack:_____

Date:_____

A.M. Glucose Reading:_____

---

Breakfast:

Time:_____    Total Carbs:_____

_____

_____

_____

Two Hour Glucose Reading:_____

Mid Morning Snack:_____

---

Lunch:

Time:_____    Total Carbs:_____

_____

_____

_____

Two Hour Glucose Reading:_____

Mid Afternoon Snack:_____

---

Dinner:

Time:_____Total Carbs:_____

_____

_____

_____

Two Hour Glucose Reading:_____

Evening Snack:_____

Date:_____

A.M. Glucose Reading:_____

Breakfast:

Time:_____  Total Carbs:_____

_____
_____
_____

Two Hour Glucose Reading:_____
Mid Morning Snack:_____

Lunch:

Time:_____  Total Carbs:_____

_____
_____
_____

Two Hour Glucose Reading:_____
Mid Afternoon Snack:_____

Dinner:

Time:_____Total Carbs:_____

_____
_____
_____

Two Hour Glucose Reading:_____
Evening Snack:_____

Date:_____

A.M. Glucose Reading:_____

Breakfast:

Time:_____ Total Carbs:_____

_____
_____
_____

Two Hour Glucose Reading:_____
Mid Morning Snack:_____

Lunch:

Time:_____ Total Carbs:_____

_____
_____
_____

Two Hour Glucose Reading:_____
Mid Afternoon Snack:_____

Dinner:

Time:_____Total Carbs:_____

_____
_____
_____

Two Hour Glucose Reading:_____
Evening Snack:_____

Date:_____

A.M. Glucose Reading:_____

Breakfast:

Time:_____ Total Carbs:_____

_____

_____

_____

Two Hour Glucose Reading:_____

Mid Morning Snack:_____

Lunch:

Time:_____ Total Carbs:_____

_____

_____

_____

Two Hour Glucose Reading:_____

Mid Afternoon Snack:_____

Dinner:

Time:_____Total Carbs:_____

_____

_____

_____

Two Hour Glucose Reading:_____

Evening Snack:_____

Date:_____

A.M. Glucose Reading:_____

Breakfast:

Time:_____ Total Carbs:_____

_____

_____

_____

Two Hour Glucose Reading:_____

Mid Morning Snack:_____

Lunch:

Time:_____ Total Carbs:_____

_____

_____

_____

Two Hour Glucose Reading:_____

Mid Afternoon Snack:_____

Dinner:

Time:_____Total Carbs:_____

_____

_____

_____

Two Hour Glucose Reading:_____

Evening Snack:_____

Date:_____

A.M. Glucose Reading:_____

---

Breakfast:

Time:_____  Total Carbs:_____

_____

_____

_____

Two Hour Glucose Reading:_____

Mid Morning Snack:_____

---

Lunch:

Time:_____  Total Carbs:_____

_____

_____

_____

Two Hour Glucose Reading:_____

Mid Afternoon Snack:_____

---

Dinner:

Time:_____Total Carbs:_____

_____

_____

_____

Two Hour Glucose Reading:_____

Evening Snack:_____

Date:_____

A.M. Glucose Reading:_____

Breakfast:

Time:_____ Total Carbs:_____

_____
_____
_____

Two Hour Glucose Reading:_____
Mid Morning Snack:_____

Lunch:

Time:_____ Total Carbs:_____

_____
_____
_____

Two Hour Glucose Reading:_____
Mid Afternoon Snack:_____

Dinner:

Time:_____Total Carbs:_____

_____
_____
_____

Two Hour Glucose Reading:_____
Evening Snack:_____

Date:_____

A.M. Glucose Reading:_____

Breakfast:

Time:_____ Total Carbs:_____

_____
_____
_____

Two Hour Glucose Reading:_____
Mid Morning Snack:_____

Lunch:

Time:_____ Total Carbs:_____

_____
_____
_____

Two Hour Glucose Reading:_____
Mid Afternoon Snack:_____

Dinner:

Time:_____Total Carbs:_____

_____
_____
_____

Two Hour Glucose Reading:_____
Evening Snack:_____

Date:_____

A.M. Glucose Reading:_____

Breakfast:

Time:_____ Total Carbs:_____
_____
_____
_____

Two Hour Glucose Reading:_____
Mid Morning Snack:_____

Lunch:

Time:_____ Total Carbs:_____
_____
_____
_____

Two Hour Glucose Reading:_____
Mid Afternoon Snack:_____

Dinner:

Time:_____ Total Carbs:_____
_____
_____
_____

Two Hour Glucose Reading:_____
Evening Snack:_____

Date:_____

A.M. Glucose Reading:_____

---

Breakfast:

Time:_____ Total Carbs:_____

_____

_____

_____

Two Hour Glucose Reading:_____

Mid Morning Snack:_____

---

Lunch:

Time:_____ Total Carbs:_____

_____

_____

_____

Two Hour Glucose Reading:_____

Mid Afternoon Snack:_____

---

Dinner:

Time:_____Total Carbs:_____

_____

_____

_____

Two Hour Glucose Reading:_____

Evening Snack:_____

Date:_____

A.M. Glucose Reading:_____

Breakfast:

Time:_____  Total Carbs:_____

_____
_____
_____

Two Hour Glucose Reading:_____
Mid Morning Snack:_____

Lunch:

Time:_____  Total Carbs:_____

_____
_____
_____

Two Hour Glucose Reading:_____
Mid Afternoon Snack:_____

Dinner:

Time:_____Total Carbs:_____

_____
_____
_____

Two Hour Glucose Reading:_____
Evening Snack:_____

Date:_____

A.M. Glucose Reading:_____

---

Breakfast:

Time:_____ Total Carbs:_____

_____
_____
_____

Two Hour Glucose Reading:_____
Mid Morning Snack:_____

---

Lunch:

Time:_____ Total Carbs:_____

_____
_____
_____

Two Hour Glucose Reading:_____
Mid Afternoon Snack:_____

---

Dinner:

Time:_____Total Carbs:_____

_____
_____
_____

Two Hour Glucose Reading:_____
Evening Snack:_____

Date:_____

A.M. Glucose Reading:_____

Breakfast:

Time:_____ Total Carbs:_____

_____
_____
_____

Two Hour Glucose Reading:_____
Mid Morning Snack:_____

Lunch:

Time:_____ Total Carbs:_____

_____
_____
_____

Two Hour Glucose Reading:_____
Mid Afternoon Snack:_____

Dinner:

Time:_____Total Carbs:_____

_____
_____
_____

Two Hour Glucose Reading:_____
Evening Snack:_____

Date:_____

A.M. Glucose Reading:_____

Breakfast:

Time:_____ Total Carbs:_____

_____

_____

_____

Two Hour Glucose Reading:_____

Mid Morning Snack:_____

Lunch:

Time:_____ Total Carbs:_____

_____

_____

_____

Two Hour Glucose Reading:_____

Mid Afternoon Snack:_____

Dinner:

Time:_____Total Carbs:_____

_____

_____

_____

Two Hour Glucose Reading:_____

Evening Snack:_____

Date:_____

A.M. Glucose Reading:_____

Breakfast:

Time:_____ Total Carbs:_____

_____
_____
_____

Two Hour Glucose Reading:_____
Mid Morning Snack:_____

Lunch:

Time:_____ Total Carbs:_____

_____
_____
_____

Two Hour Glucose Reading:_____
Mid Afternoon Snack:_____

Dinner:

Time:_____Total Carbs:_____

_____
_____
_____

Two Hour Glucose Reading:_____
Evening Snack:_____

Date:_____

A.M. Glucose Reading:_____

---

Breakfast:

Time:_____ Total Carbs:_____

_____

_____

_____

Two Hour Glucose Reading:_____

Mid Morning Snack:_____

---

Lunch:

Time:_____ Total Carbs:_____

_____

_____

_____

Two Hour Glucose Reading:_____

Mid Afternoon Snack:_____

---

Dinner:

Time:_____Total Carbs:_____

_____

_____

_____

Two Hour Glucose Reading:_____

Evening Snack:_____

Date:_____

A.M. Glucose Reading:_____

Breakfast:

Time:_____ Total Carbs:_____
_____
_____
_____
Two Hour Glucose Reading:_____
Mid Morning Snack:_____

Lunch:

Time:_____ Total Carbs:_____
_____
_____
_____
Two Hour Glucose Reading:_____
Mid Afternoon Snack:_____

Dinner:

Time:_____Total Carbs:_____
_____
_____
_____
Two Hour Glucose Reading:_____
Evening Snack:_____

Date:_____

A.M. Glucose Reading:_____

Breakfast:

Time:_____ Total Carbs:_____
_____
_____
_____

Two Hour Glucose Reading:_____
Mid Morning Snack:_____

Lunch:

Time:_____ Total Carbs:_____
_____
_____
_____

Two Hour Glucose Reading:_____
Mid Afternoon Snack:_____

Dinner:

Time:_____Total Carbs:_____
_____
_____
_____

Two Hour Glucose Reading:_____
Evening Snack:_____

Date:_____

A.M. Glucose Reading:_____

---

Breakfast:

Time:_____ Total Carbs:_____
_____
_____
_____

Two Hour Glucose Reading:_____
Mid Morning Snack:_____

---

Lunch:

Time:_____ Total Carbs:_____
_____
_____
_____

Two Hour Glucose Reading:_____
Mid Afternoon Snack:_____

---

Dinner:

Time:_____Total Carbs:_____
_____
_____
_____

Two Hour Glucose Reading:_____
Evening Snack:_____

Date:_____

A.M. Glucose Reading:_____

Breakfast:

Time:_____ Total Carbs:_____

_____

_____

_____

Two Hour Glucose Reading:_____

Mid Morning Snack:_____

Lunch:

Time:_____ Total Carbs:_____

_____

_____

_____

Two Hour Glucose Reading:_____

Mid Afternoon Snack:_____

Dinner:

Time:_____Total Carbs:_____

_____

_____

_____

Two Hour Glucose Reading:_____

Evening Snack:_____

Date:_____

A.M. Glucose Reading:_____

Breakfast:

Time:_____ Total Carbs:_____

_____

_____

_____

Two Hour Glucose Reading:_____

Mid Morning Snack:_____

Lunch:

Time:_____ Total Carbs:_____

_____

_____

_____

Two Hour Glucose Reading:_____

Mid Afternoon Snack:_____

Dinner:

Time:_____Total Carbs:_____

_____

_____

_____

Two Hour Glucose Reading:_____

Evening Snack:_____

Date:_____

A.M. Glucose Reading:_____

Breakfast:

Time:_____ Total Carbs:_____

_____
_____
_____

Two Hour Glucose Reading:_____
Mid Morning Snack:_____

Lunch:

Time:_____ Total Carbs:_____

_____
_____
_____

Two Hour Glucose Reading:_____
Mid Afternoon Snack:_____

Dinner:

Time:_____Total Carbs:_____

_____
_____
_____

Two Hour Glucose Reading:_____
Evening Snack:_____

Date:_____

A.M. Glucose Reading:_____

Breakfast:

Time:_____  Total Carbs:_____

_____

_____

_____

Two Hour Glucose Reading:_____

Mid Morning Snack:_____

Lunch:

Time:_____  Total Carbs:_____

_____

_____

_____

Two Hour Glucose Reading:_____

Mid Afternoon Snack:_____

Dinner:

Time:_____Total Carbs:_____

_____

_____

_____

Two Hour Glucose Reading:_____

Evening Snack:_____

Date:_____

A.M. Glucose Reading:_____

Breakfast:

Time:_____ Total Carbs:_____

_____
_____
_____

Two Hour Glucose Reading:_____
Mid Morning Snack:_____

Lunch:

Time:_____ Total Carbs:_____

_____
_____
_____

Two Hour Glucose Reading:_____
Mid Afternoon Snack:_____

Dinner:

Time:_____Total Carbs:_____

_____
_____
_____

Two Hour Glucose Reading:_____
Evening Snack:_____

Date:_____

A.M. Glucose Reading:_____

Breakfast:

Time:_____   Total Carbs:_____

_____

_____

_____

Two Hour Glucose Reading:_____

Mid Morning Snack:_____

Lunch:

Time:_____   Total Carbs:_____

_____

_____

_____

Two Hour Glucose Reading:_____
Mid Afternoon Snack:_____

Dinner:

Time:_____   Total Carbs:_____

_____

_____

_____

Two Hour Glucose Reading:_____
Evening Snack:_____

Date:_____

A.M. Glucose Reading:_____

Breakfast:

Time:_____ Total Carbs:_____

_____
_____
_____

Two Hour Glucose Reading:_____
Mid Morning Snack:_____

Lunch:

Time:_____ Total Carbs:_____

_____
_____
_____

Two Hour Glucose Reading:_____
Mid Afternoon Snack:_____

Dinner:

Time:_____Total Carbs:_____

_____
_____
_____

Two Hour Glucose Reading:_____
Evening Snack:_____

Date:_____

A.M. Glucose Reading:_____

---

Breakfast:

Time:_____ Total Carbs:_____
_____
_____
_____

Two Hour Glucose Reading:_____
Mid Morning Snack:_____

---

Lunch:

Time:_____ Total Carbs:_____
_____
_____
_____

Two Hour Glucose Reading:_____
Mid Afternoon Snack:_____

---

Dinner:

Time:_____Total Carbs:_____
_____
_____
_____

Two Hour Glucose Reading:_____
Evening Snack:_____

Date:_____

A.M. Glucose Reading:_____

Breakfast:

Time:_____  Total Carbs:_____

_____
_____
_____

Two Hour Glucose Reading:_____
Mid Morning Snack:_____

Lunch:

Time:_____  Total Carbs:_____

_____
_____
_____

Two Hour Glucose Reading:_____
Mid Afternoon Snack:_____

Dinner:

Time:_____  Total Carbs:_____

_____
_____
_____

Two Hour Glucose Reading:_____
Evening Snack:_____

Date:_____

A.M. Glucose Reading:_____

Breakfast:

Time:_____ Total Carbs:_____

_____
_____
_____

Two Hour Glucose Reading:_____
Mid Morning Snack:_____

Lunch:

Time:_____ Total Carbs:_____

_____
_____
_____

Two Hour Glucose Reading:_____
Mid Afternoon Snack:_____

Dinner:

Time:_____Total Carbs:_____

_____
_____
_____

Two Hour Glucose Reading:_____
Evening Snack:_____

Date:_____

A.M. Glucose Reading:_____

Breakfast:

Time:_____ Total Carbs:_____

_____

_____

_____

Two Hour Glucose Reading:_____

Mid Morning Snack:_____

Lunch:

Time:_____ Total Carbs:_____

_____

_____

_____

Two Hour Glucose Reading:_____

Mid Afternoon Snack:_____

Dinner:

Time:_____Total Carbs:_____

_____

_____

_____

Two Hour Glucose Reading:_____

Evening Snack:_____

Date:_____

A.M. Glucose Reading:_____

Breakfast:

Time:_____ Total Carbs:_____
_____
_____
_____

Two Hour Glucose Reading:_____
Mid Morning Snack:_____

Lunch:

Time:_____ Total Carbs:_____
_____
_____
_____

Two Hour Glucose Reading:_____
Mid Afternoon Snack:_____

Dinner:

Time:_____Total Carbs:_____
_____
_____
_____

Two Hour Glucose Reading:_____
Evening Snack:_____

Date:_____

A.M. Glucose Reading:_____

Breakfast:

Time:_____ Total Carbs:_____

_____
_____
_____

Two Hour Glucose Reading:_____
Mid Morning Snack:_____

Lunch:

Time:_____ Total Carbs:_____

_____
_____
_____

Two Hour Glucose Reading:_____
Mid Afternoon Snack:_____

Dinner:

Time:_____Total Carbs:_____

_____
_____
_____

Two Hour Glucose Reading:_____
Evening Snack:_____

Date:_____

A.M. Glucose Reading:_____

Breakfast:

Time:_____ Total Carbs:_____

_____
_____
_____

Two Hour Glucose Reading:_____
Mid Morning Snack:_____

Lunch:

Time:_____ Total Carbs:_____

_____
_____
_____

Two Hour Glucose Reading:_____
Mid Afternoon Snack:_____

Dinner:

Time:_____ Total Carbs:_____

_____
_____
_____

Two Hour Glucose Reading:_____
Evening Snack:_____

Date:_____

A.M. Glucose Reading:_____

Breakfast:

Time:_____ Total Carbs:_____

_____
_____
_____

Two Hour Glucose Reading:_____
Mid Morning Snack:_____

Lunch:

Time:_____ Total Carbs:_____

_____
_____
_____

Two Hour Glucose Reading:_____
Mid Afternoon Snack:_____

Dinner:

Time:_____Total Carbs:_____

_____
_____
_____

Two Hour Glucose Reading:_____
Evening Snack:_____

Date:_____

A.M. Glucose Reading:_____

Breakfast:

Time:_____    Total Carbs:_____

_____

_____

_____

Two Hour Glucose Reading:_____

Mid Morning Snack:_____

---

Lunch:

Time:_____    Total Carbs:_____

_____

_____

_____

Two Hour Glucose Reading:_____

Mid Afternoon Snack:_____

---

Dinner:

Time:_____    Total Carbs:_____

_____

_____

_____

Two Hour Glucose Reading:_____

Evening Snack:_____

Date:_____

A.M. Glucose Reading:_____

Breakfast:

Time:_____ Total Carbs:_____

_____
_____
_____

Two Hour Glucose Reading:_____

Mid Morning Snack:_____

Lunch:

Time:_____ Total Carbs:_____

_____
_____
_____

Two Hour Glucose Reading:_____
Mid Afternoon Snack:_____

Dinner:

Time:_____Total Carbs:_____

_____
_____
_____

Two Hour Glucose Reading:_____
Evening Snack:_____

Date:_____

A.M. Glucose Reading:_____

Breakfast:

Time:_____ Total Carbs:_____

_____
_____
_____

Two Hour Glucose Reading:_____
Mid Morning Snack:_____

Lunch:

Time:_____ Total Carbs:_____

_____
_____
_____

Two Hour Glucose Reading:_____
Mid Afternoon Snack:_____

Dinner:

Time:_____Total Carbs:_____

_____
_____
_____

Two Hour Glucose Reading:_____
Evening Snack:_____

Date:_____

A.M. Glucose Reading:_____

---

Breakfast:

Time:_____  Total Carbs:_____

_____

_____

_____

Two Hour Glucose Reading:_____

Mid Morning Snack:_____

---

Lunch:

Time:_____  Total Carbs:_____

_____

_____

_____

Two Hour Glucose Reading:_____

Mid Afternoon Snack:_____

---

Dinner:

Time:_____Total Carbs:_____

_____

_____

_____

Two Hour Glucose Reading:_____

Evening Snack:_____

Date:_____

A.M. Glucose Reading:_____

Breakfast:

Time:_____     Total Carbs:_____
_____
_____
_____

Two Hour Glucose Reading:_____
Mid Morning Snack:_____

Lunch:

Time:_____     Total Carbs:_____
_____
_____
_____

Two Hour Glucose Reading:_____
Mid Afternoon Snack:_____

Dinner:

Time:_____Total Carbs:_____
_____
_____
_____

Two Hour Glucose Reading:_____
Evening Snack:_____

Date:_____

A.M. Glucose Reading:_____

Breakfast:

Time:_____ Total Carbs:_____

_____
_____
_____

Two Hour Glucose Reading:_____
Mid Morning Snack:_____

Lunch:

Time:_____ Total Carbs:_____

_____
_____
_____

Two Hour Glucose Reading:_____
Mid Afternoon Snack:_____

Dinner:

Time:_____Total Carbs:_____

_____
_____
_____

Two Hour Glucose Reading:_____
Evening Snack:_____

Date:_____

A.M. Glucose Reading:_____

Breakfast:

Time:_____  Total Carbs:_____

_____
_____
_____

Two Hour Glucose Reading:_____
Mid Morning Snack:_____

Lunch:

Time:_____  Total Carbs:_____

_____
_____
_____

Two Hour Glucose Reading:_____
Mid Afternoon Snack:_____

Dinner:

Time:_____  Total Carbs:_____

_____
_____
_____

Two Hour Glucose Reading:_____
Evening Snack:_____

Date:_____

A.M. Glucose Reading:_____

Breakfast:

Time:_____ Total Carbs:_____

_____

_____

_____

Two Hour Glucose Reading:_____

Mid Morning Snack:_____

Lunch:

Time:_____ Total Carbs:_____

_____

_____

_____

Two Hour Glucose Reading:_____

Mid Afternoon Snack:_____

Dinner:

Time:_____Total Carbs:_____

_____

_____

_____

Two Hour Glucose Reading:_____

Evening Snack:_____

Date:_____

A.M. Glucose Reading:_____

Breakfast:

Time:_____ Total Carbs:_____
_____
_____
_____

Two Hour Glucose Reading:_____
Mid Morning Snack:_____

Lunch:

Time:_____ Total Carbs:_____
_____
_____
_____

Two Hour Glucose Reading:_____
Mid Afternoon Snack:_____

Dinner:

Time:_____Total Carbs:_____
_____
_____
_____

Two Hour Glucose Reading:_____
Evening Snack:_____

Date:_____

A.M. Glucose Reading:_____

---

Breakfast:

Time:_____ Total Carbs:_____
_____
_____
_____

Two Hour Glucose Reading:_____
Mid Morning Snack:_____

---

Lunch:

Time:_____ Total Carbs:_____
_____
_____
_____

Two Hour Glucose Reading:_____
Mid Afternoon Snack:_____

---

Dinner:

Time:_____Total Carbs:_____
_____
_____
_____

Two Hour Glucose Reading:_____
Evening Snack:_____

Date:_____

A.M. Glucose Reading:_____

---

Breakfast:

Time:_____  Total Carbs:_____

_____

_____

_____

Two Hour Glucose Reading:_____

Mid Morning Snack:_____

---

Lunch:

Time:_____  Total Carbs:_____

_____

_____

_____

Two Hour Glucose Reading:_____

Mid Afternoon Snack:_____

---

Dinner:

Time:_____Total Carbs:_____

_____

_____

_____

Two Hour Glucose Reading:_____

Evening Snack:_____

Date:_____

A.M. Glucose Reading:_____

Breakfast:

Time:_____ Total Carbs:_____

_____

_____

_____

Two Hour Glucose Reading:_____

Mid Morning Snack:_____

Lunch:

Time:_____ Total Carbs:_____

_____

_____

_____

Two Hour Glucose Reading:_____

Mid Afternoon Snack:_____

Dinner:

Time:_____Total Carbs:_____

_____

_____

_____

Two Hour Glucose Reading:_____

Evening Snack:_____

Date:_____

A.M. Glucose Reading:_____

Breakfast:

Time:_____ Total Carbs:_____

_____
_____
_____

Two Hour Glucose Reading:_____
Mid Morning Snack:_____

Lunch:

Time:_____ Total Carbs:_____

_____
_____
_____

Two Hour Glucose Reading:_____
Mid Afternoon Snack:_____

Dinner:

Time:_____Total Carbs:_____

_____
_____
_____

Two Hour Glucose Reading:_____
Evening Snack:_____

Date:_____

A.M. Glucose Reading:_____

Breakfast:

Time:_____    Total Carbs:_____

_____

_____

_____

Two Hour Glucose Reading:_____

Mid Morning Snack:_____

Lunch:

Time:_____    Total Carbs:_____

_____

_____

_____

Two Hour Glucose Reading:_____

Mid Afternoon Snack:_____

Dinner:

Time:_____Total Carbs:_____

_____

_____

_____

Two Hour Glucose Reading:_____

Evening Snack:_____

Date:_____

A.M. Glucose Reading:_____

Breakfast:

Time:_____  Total Carbs:_____

_____
_____
_____

Two Hour Glucose Reading:_____
Mid Morning Snack:_____

Lunch:

Time:_____  Total Carbs:_____

_____
_____
_____

Two Hour Glucose Reading:_____
Mid Afternoon Snack:_____

Dinner:

Time:_____Total Carbs:_____

_____
_____
_____

Two Hour Glucose Reading:_____
Evening Snack:_____

Date:_____

A.M. Glucose Reading:_____

Breakfast:

Time:_____ Total Carbs:_____
_____
_____
_____

Two Hour Glucose Reading:_____
Mid Morning Snack:_____

Lunch:

Time:_____ Total Carbs:_____
_____
_____
_____

Two Hour Glucose Reading:_____
Mid Afternoon Snack:_____

Dinner:

Time:_____Total Carbs:_____
_____
_____
_____

Two Hour Glucose Reading:_____
Evening Snack:_____

Date:_____

A.M. Glucose Reading:_____

Breakfast:

Time:_____    Total Carbs:_____

_____

_____

_____

Two Hour Glucose Reading:_____

Mid Morning Snack:_____

Lunch:

Time:_____    Total Carbs:_____

_____

_____

_____

Two Hour Glucose Reading:_____

Mid Afternoon Snack:_____

Dinner:

Time:_____Total Carbs:_____

_____

_____

_____

Two Hour Glucose Reading:_____

Evening Snack:_____

Date:_____

A.M. Glucose Reading:_____

Breakfast:

Time:_____ Total Carbs:_____
_____
_____
_____

Two Hour Glucose Reading:_____
Mid Morning Snack:_____

Lunch:

Time:_____ Total Carbs:_____
_____
_____
_____

Two Hour Glucose Reading:_____
Mid Afternoon Snack:_____

Dinner:

Time:_____Total Carbs:_____
_____
_____
_____

Two Hour Glucose Reading:_____
Evening Snack:_____

Date:_____

A.M. Glucose Reading:_____

Breakfast:

Time:_____    Total Carbs:_____
_____
_____
_____

Two Hour Glucose Reading:_____
Mid Morning Snack:_____

Lunch:

Time:_____    Total Carbs:_____
_____
_____
_____

Two Hour Glucose Reading:_____
Mid Afternoon Snack:_____

Dinner:

Time:_____    Total Carbs:_____
_____
_____
_____

Two Hour Glucose Reading:_____
Evening Snack:_____

Date:_____

A.M. Glucose Reading:_____

Breakfast:

Time:_____ Total Carbs:_____

_____

_____

_____

Two Hour Glucose Reading:_____

Mid Morning Snack:_____

Lunch:

Time:_____ Total Carbs:_____

_____

_____

_____

Two Hour Glucose Reading:_____

Mid Afternoon Snack:_____

Dinner:

Time:_____Total Carbs:_____

_____

_____

_____

Two Hour Glucose Reading:_____

Evening Snack:_____

Date:_____

A.M. Glucose Reading:_____

Breakfast:

Time:_____ Total Carbs:_____
_____
_____
_____

Two Hour Glucose Reading:_____
Mid Morning Snack:_____

Lunch:

Time:_____ Total Carbs:_____
_____
_____
_____

Two Hour Glucose Reading:_____
Mid Afternoon Snack:_____

Dinner:

Time:_____Total Carbs:_____
_____
_____
_____

Two Hour Glucose Reading:_____
Evening Snack:_____

Date:_____

A.M. Glucose Reading:_____

Breakfast:

Time:_____ Total Carbs:_____

_____
_____
_____

Two Hour Glucose Reading:_____
Mid Morning Snack:_____

Lunch:

Time:_____ Total Carbs:_____

_____
_____
_____

Two Hour Glucose Reading:_____
Mid Afternoon Snack:_____

Dinner:

Time:_____Total Carbs:_____

_____
_____
_____

Two Hour Glucose Reading:_____
Evening Snack:_____

Date:_____

A.M. Glucose Reading:_____

Breakfast:

Time:_____    Total Carbs:_____

_____

_____

_____

Two Hour Glucose Reading:_____

Mid Morning Snack:_____

Lunch:

Time:_____    Total Carbs:_____

_____

_____

_____

Two Hour Glucose Reading:_____

Mid Afternoon Snack:_____

Dinner:

Time:_____    Total Carbs:_____

_____

_____

_____

Two Hour Glucose Reading:_____

Evening Snack:_____

Date:_____

A.M. Glucose Reading:_____

---

**Breakfast:**

Time:_____   Total Carbs:_____

_____

_____

_____

Two Hour Glucose Reading:_____

Mid Morning Snack:_____

---

**Lunch:**

Time:_____   Total Carbs:_____

_____

_____

_____

Two Hour Glucose Reading:_____

Mid Afternoon Snack:_____

---

**Dinner:**

Time:_____Total Carbs:_____

_____

_____

_____

Two Hour Glucose Reading:_____

Evening Snack:_____

Date:_____

A.M. Glucose Reading:_____

Breakfast:

Time:_____ Total Carbs:_____

_____
_____
_____

Two Hour Glucose Reading:_____
Mid Morning Snack:_____

Lunch:

Time:_____ Total Carbs:_____

_____
_____
_____

Two Hour Glucose Reading:_____
Mid Afternoon Snack:_____

Dinner:

Time:_____Total Carbs:_____

_____
_____
_____

Two Hour Glucose Reading:_____
Evening Snack:_____

Date:_____

A.M. Glucose Reading:_____

Breakfast:

Time:_____ Total Carbs:_____
_____
_____
_____

Two Hour Glucose Reading:_____
Mid Morning Snack:_____

Lunch:

Time:_____ Total Carbs:_____
_____
_____
_____

Two Hour Glucose Reading:_____
Mid Afternoon Snack:_____

Dinner:

Time:_____Total Carbs:_____
_____
_____
_____

Two Hour Glucose Reading:_____
Evening Snack:_____

Date:_____

A.M. Glucose Reading:_____

Breakfast:

Time:_____  Total Carbs:_____

_____

_____

_____

Two Hour Glucose Reading:_____

Mid Morning Snack:_____

Lunch:

Time:_____  Total Carbs:_____

_____

_____

_____

Two Hour Glucose Reading:_____

Mid Afternoon Snack:_____

Dinner:

Time:_____  Total Carbs:_____

_____

_____

_____

Two Hour Glucose Reading:_____

Evening Snack:_____

Date:_____

A.M. Glucose Reading:_____

Breakfast:

Time:_____ Total Carbs:_____

_____

_____

_____

Two Hour Glucose Reading:_____

Mid Morning Snack:_____

Lunch:

Time:_____ Total Carbs:_____

_____

_____

_____

Two Hour Glucose Reading:_____

Mid Afternoon Snack:_____

Dinner:

Time:_____Total Carbs:_____

_____

_____

_____

Two Hour Glucose Reading:_____

Evening Snack:_____

Date:_____

A.M. Glucose Reading:_____

Breakfast:

Time:_____ Total Carbs:_____
_____
_____
_____

Two Hour Glucose Reading:_____
Mid Morning Snack:_____

Lunch:

Time:_____ Total Carbs:_____
_____
_____
_____

Two Hour Glucose Reading:_____
Mid Afternoon Snack:_____

Dinner:

Time:_____Total Carbs:_____
_____
_____
_____

Two Hour Glucose Reading:_____
Evening Snack:_____

Date:_____

A.M. Glucose Reading:_____

Breakfast:

Time:_____ Total Carbs:_____

_____

_____

_____

Two Hour Glucose Reading:_____

Mid Morning Snack:_____

Lunch:

Time:_____ Total Carbs:_____

_____

_____

_____

Two Hour Glucose Reading:_____

Mid Afternoon Snack:_____

Dinner:

Time:_____Total Carbs:_____

_____

_____

_____

Two Hour Glucose Reading:_____

Evening Snack:_____

Date:_____

A.M. Glucose Reading:_____

Breakfast:

Time:_____ Total Carbs:_____

_____
_____
_____

Two Hour Glucose Reading:_____
Mid Morning Snack:_____

Lunch:

Time:_____ Total Carbs:_____

_____
_____
_____

Two Hour Glucose Reading:_____
Mid Afternoon Snack:_____

Dinner:

Time:_____ Total Carbs:_____

_____
_____
_____

Two Hour Glucose Reading:_____
Evening Snack:_____

Date:_____

A.M. Glucose Reading:_____

Breakfast:

Time:_____ Total Carbs:_____

_____

_____

_____

Two Hour Glucose Reading:_____

Mid Morning Snack:_____

Lunch:

Time:_____ Total Carbs:_____

_____

_____

_____

Two Hour Glucose Reading:_____

Mid Afternoon Snack:_____

Dinner:

Time:_____Total Carbs:_____

_____

_____

_____

Two Hour Glucose Reading:_____

Evening Snack:_____

Date:_____

A.M. Glucose Reading:_____

Breakfast:

Time:_____ Total Carbs:_____
_____
_____
_____

Two Hour Glucose Reading:_____
Mid Morning Snack:_____

Lunch:

Time:_____ Total Carbs:_____
_____
_____
_____

Two Hour Glucose Reading:_____
Mid Afternoon Snack:_____

Dinner:

Time:_____ Total Carbs:_____
_____
_____
_____

Two Hour Glucose Reading:_____
Evening Snack:_____

Date:_____

A.M. Glucose Reading:_____

Breakfast:

Time:_____ Total Carbs:_____

_____
_____
_____

Two Hour Glucose Reading:_____
Mid Morning Snack:_____

Lunch:

Time:_____ Total Carbs:_____

_____
_____
_____

Two Hour Glucose Reading:_____
Mid Afternoon Snack:_____

Dinner:

Time:_____Total Carbs:_____

_____
_____
_____

Two Hour Glucose Reading:_____
Evening Snack:_____

Date:_____

A.M. Glucose Reading:_____

Breakfast:

Time:_____ Total Carbs:_____

_____

_____

_____

Two Hour Glucose Reading:_____

Mid Morning Snack:_____

Lunch:

Time:_____ Total Carbs:_____

_____

_____

_____

Two Hour Glucose Reading:_____
Mid Afternoon Snack:_____

Dinner:

Time:_____ Total Carbs:_____

_____

_____

_____

Two Hour Glucose Reading:_____
Evening Snack:_____

Date:_____

A.M. Glucose Reading:_____

---

Breakfast:

Time:_____ Total Carbs:_____

_____
_____
_____

Two Hour Glucose Reading:_____
Mid Morning Snack:_____

---

Lunch:

Time:_____ Total Carbs:_____

_____
_____
_____

Two Hour Glucose Reading:_____
Mid Afternoon Snack:_____

---

Dinner:

Time:_____Total Carbs:_____

_____
_____
_____

Two Hour Glucose Reading:_____
Evening Snack:_____

Date:_____

A.M. Glucose Reading:_____

Breakfast:

Time:_____ Total Carbs:_____
_____
_____
_____

Two Hour Glucose Reading:_____
Mid Morning Snack:_____

Lunch:

Time:_____ Total Carbs:_____
_____
_____
_____

Two Hour Glucose Reading:_____
Mid Afternoon Snack:_____

Dinner:

Time:_____Total Carbs:_____
_____
_____
_____

Two Hour Glucose Reading:_____
Evening Snack:_____

Date:_____

A.M. Glucose Reading:_____

Breakfast:

Time:_____ Total Carbs:_____

_____
_____
_____

Two Hour Glucose Reading:_____
Mid Morning Snack:_____

Lunch:

Time:_____ Total Carbs:_____

_____
_____
_____

Two Hour Glucose Reading:_____
Mid Afternoon Snack:_____

Dinner:

Time:_____Total Carbs:_____

_____
_____
_____

Two Hour Glucose Reading:_____
Evening Snack:_____

Date:_____

A.M. Glucose Reading:_____

Breakfast:

Time:_____ Total Carbs:_____

_____
_____
_____

Two Hour Glucose Reading:_____
Mid Morning Snack:_____

Lunch:

Time:_____ Total Carbs:_____

_____
_____
_____

Two Hour Glucose Reading:_____
Mid Afternoon Snack:_____

Dinner:

Time:_____Total Carbs:_____

_____
_____
_____

Two Hour Glucose Reading:_____
Evening Snack:_____

Date:_____

A.M. Glucose Reading:_____

Breakfast:

Time:_____ Total Carbs:_____

_____
_____
_____

Two Hour Glucose Reading:_____
Mid Morning Snack:_____

Lunch:

Time:_____ Total Carbs:_____

_____
_____
_____

Two Hour Glucose Reading:_____
Mid Afternoon Snack:_____

Dinner:

Time:_____Total Carbs:_____

_____
_____
_____

Two Hour Glucose Reading:_____
Evening Snack:_____

Date:_____

A.M. Glucose Reading:_____

Breakfast:

Time:_____ Total Carbs:_____

_____

_____

_____

Two Hour Glucose Reading:_____

Mid Morning Snack:_____

Lunch:

Time:_____ Total Carbs:_____

_____

_____

_____

Two Hour Glucose Reading:_____

Mid Afternoon Snack:_____

Dinner:

Time:_____ Total Carbs:_____

_____

_____

_____

Two Hour Glucose Reading:_____

Evening Snack:_____

Date:_____

A.M. Glucose Reading:_____

Breakfast:

Time:_____    Total Carbs:_____

_____
_____
_____

Two Hour Glucose Reading:_____
Mid Morning Snack:_____

Lunch:

Time:_____    Total Carbs:_____

_____
_____
_____

Two Hour Glucose Reading:_____
Mid Afternoon Snack:_____

Dinner:

Time:_____    Total Carbs:_____

_____
_____
_____

Two Hour Glucose Reading:_____
Evening Snack:_____

Date:_____

A.M. Glucose Reading:_____

Breakfast:

Time:_____ Total Carbs:_____

_____
_____
_____

Two Hour Glucose Reading:_____
Mid Morning Snack:_____

Lunch:

Time:_____ Total Carbs:_____

_____
_____
_____

Two Hour Glucose Reading:_____
Mid Afternoon Snack:_____

Dinner:

Time:_____Total Carbs:_____

_____
_____
_____

Two Hour Glucose Reading:_____
Evening Snack:_____

Date:_____

A.M. Glucose Reading:_____

Breakfast:

Time:_____ Total Carbs:_____

_____

_____

_____

Two Hour Glucose Reading:_____

Mid Morning Snack:_____

Lunch:

Time:_____ Total Carbs:_____

_____

_____

_____

Two Hour Glucose Reading:_____

Mid Afternoon Snack:_____

Dinner:

Time:_____Total Carbs:_____

_____

_____

_____

Two Hour Glucose Reading:_____

Evening Snack:_____

Date:_____

A.M. Glucose Reading:_____

Breakfast:

Time:_____     Total Carbs:_____

_____

_____

_____

Two Hour Glucose Reading:_____

Mid Morning Snack:_____

Lunch:

Time:_____     Total Carbs:_____

_____

_____

_____

Two Hour Glucose Reading:_____

Mid Afternoon Snack:_____

Dinner:

Time:_____Total Carbs:_____

_____

_____

_____

Two Hour Glucose Reading:_____

Evening Snack:_____

Date:_____

A.M. Glucose Reading:_____

Breakfast:

Time:_____ Total Carbs:_____

_____

_____

_____

Two Hour Glucose Reading:_____

Mid Morning Snack:_____

Lunch:

Time:_____ Total Carbs:_____

_____

_____

_____

Two Hour Glucose Reading:_____

Mid Afternoon Snack:_____

Dinner:

Time:_____Total Carbs:_____

_____

_____

_____

Two Hour Glucose Reading:_____

Evening Snack:_____

Date:_____

A.M. Glucose Reading:_____

---

Breakfast:

Time:_____ Total Carbs:_____

_____

_____

_____

Two Hour Glucose Reading:_____

Mid Morning Snack:_____

---

Lunch:

Time:_____ Total Carbs:_____

_____

_____

_____

Two Hour Glucose Reading:_____

Mid Afternoon Snack:_____

---

Dinner:

Time:_____Total Carbs:_____

_____

_____

_____

Two Hour Glucose Reading:_____

Evening Snack:_____

Date:_____

A.M. Glucose Reading:_____

Breakfast:

Time:_____ Total Carbs:_____

_____
_____
_____

Two Hour Glucose Reading:_____
Mid Morning Snack:_____

Lunch:

Time:_____ Total Carbs:_____

_____
_____
_____

Two Hour Glucose Reading:_____
Mid Afternoon Snack:_____

Dinner:

Time:_____Total Carbs:_____

_____
_____
_____

Two Hour Glucose Reading:_____
Evening Snack:_____

Date:_____

A.M. Glucose Reading:_____

Breakfast:

Time:_____ Total Carbs:_____

_____
_____
_____

Two Hour Glucose Reading:_____
Mid Morning Snack:_____

Lunch:

Time:_____ Total Carbs:_____

_____
_____
_____

Two Hour Glucose Reading:_____
Mid Afternoon Snack:_____

Dinner:

Time:_____Total Carbs:_____

_____
_____
_____

Two Hour Glucose Reading:_____
Evening Snack:_____

Date:_____

A.M. Glucose Reading:_____

Breakfast:

Time:_____ Total Carbs:_____

_____

_____

_____

Two Hour Glucose Reading:_____

Mid Morning Snack:_____

Lunch:

Time:_____ Total Carbs:_____

_____

_____

_____

Two Hour Glucose Reading:_____

Mid Afternoon Snack:_____

Dinner:

Time:_____Total Carbs:_____

_____

_____

_____

Two Hour Glucose Reading:_____

Evening Snack:_____

Date:_____

A.M. Glucose Reading:_____

Breakfast:

Time:_____    Total Carbs:_____

_____
_____
_____

Two Hour Glucose Reading:_____
Mid Morning Snack:_____

Lunch:

Time:_____    Total Carbs:_____

_____
_____
_____

Two Hour Glucose Reading:_____
Mid Afternoon Snack:_____

Dinner:

Time:_____    Total Carbs:_____

_____
_____
_____

Two Hour Glucose Reading:_____
Evening Snack:_____

Date:_____

A.M. Glucose Reading:_____

Breakfast:

Time:_____     Total Carbs:_____

_____

_____

_____

Two Hour Glucose Reading:_____

Mid Morning Snack:_____

Lunch:

Time:_____     Total Carbs:_____

_____

_____

_____

Two Hour Glucose Reading:_____

Mid Afternoon Snack:_____

Dinner:

Time:_____Total Carbs:_____

_____

_____

_____

Two Hour Glucose Reading:_____

Evening Snack:_____

Date:_____

A.M. Glucose Reading:_____

Breakfast:

Time:_____ Total Carbs:_____
_____
_____
_____
Two Hour Glucose Reading:_____
Mid Morning Snack:_____

Lunch:

Time:_____ Total Carbs:_____
_____
_____
_____
Two Hour Glucose Reading:_____
Mid Afternoon Snack:_____

Dinner:

Time:_____Total Carbs:_____
_____
_____
_____
Two Hour Glucose Reading:_____
Evening Snack:_____

Date:_____

A.M. Glucose Reading:_____

Breakfast:

Time:_____ Total Carbs:_____

_____
_____
_____

Two Hour Glucose Reading:_____
Mid Morning Snack:_____

Lunch:

Time:_____ Total Carbs:_____

_____
_____
_____

Two Hour Glucose Reading:_____
Mid Afternoon Snack:_____

Dinner:

Time:_____Total Carbs:_____

_____
_____
_____

Two Hour Glucose Reading:_____
Evening Snack:_____

Date:_____

A.M. Glucose Reading:_____

Breakfast:

Time:_____ Total Carbs:_____

_____
_____
_____

Two Hour Glucose Reading:_____
Mid Morning Snack:_____

Lunch:

Time:_____ Total Carbs:_____

_____
_____
_____

Two Hour Glucose Reading:_____
Mid Afternoon Snack:_____

Dinner:

Time:_____ Total Carbs:_____

_____
_____
_____

Two Hour Glucose Reading:_____
Evening Snack:_____

Date:_____

A.M. Glucose Reading:_____

Breakfast:

Time:_____  Total Carbs:_____

_____
_____
_____

Two Hour Glucose Reading:_____
Mid Morning Snack:_____

Lunch:

Time:_____  Total Carbs:_____

_____
_____
_____

Two Hour Glucose Reading:_____
Mid Afternoon Snack:_____

Dinner:

Time:_____Total Carbs:_____

_____
_____
_____

Two Hour Glucose Reading:_____
Evening Snack:_____

Date:_____

A.M. Glucose Reading:_____

Breakfast:

Time:_____    Total Carbs:_____

_____
_____
_____

Two Hour Glucose Reading:_____
Mid Morning Snack:_____

Lunch:

Time:_____    Total Carbs:_____

_____
_____
_____

Two Hour Glucose Reading:_____
Mid Afternoon Snack:_____

Dinner:

Time:_____Total Carbs:_____

_____
_____
_____

Two Hour Glucose Reading:_____
Evening Snack:_____

Date:_____

A.M. Glucose Reading:_____

Breakfast:

Time:_____ Total Carbs:_____

_____
_____
_____

Two Hour Glucose Reading:_____
Mid Morning Snack:_____

Lunch:

Time:_____ Total Carbs:_____

_____
_____
_____

Two Hour Glucose Reading:_____
Mid Afternoon Snack:_____

Dinner:

Time:_____Total Carbs:_____

_____
_____
_____

Two Hour Glucose Reading:_____
Evening Snack:_____

Date:_____

A.M. Glucose Reading:_____

Breakfast:

Time:_____ Total Carbs:_____

_____

_____

_____

Two Hour Glucose Reading:_____

Mid Morning Snack:_____

Lunch:

Time:_____ Total Carbs:_____

_____

_____

_____

Two Hour Glucose Reading:_____

Mid Afternoon Snack:_____

Dinner:

Time:_____Total Carbs:_____

_____

_____

_____

Two Hour Glucose Reading:_____

Evening Snack:_____

Date:_____

A.M. Glucose Reading:_____

Breakfast:

Time:_____  Total Carbs:_____

_____

_____

_____

Two Hour Glucose Reading:_____

Mid Morning Snack:_____

Lunch:

Time:_____  Total Carbs:_____

_____

_____

_____

Two Hour Glucose Reading:_____

Mid Afternoon Snack:_____

Dinner:

Time:_____Total Carbs:_____

_____

_____

_____

Two Hour Glucose Reading:_____

Evening Snack:_____

Date:_____

A.M. Glucose Reading:_____

Breakfast:

Time:_____ Total Carbs:_____

_____

_____

_____

Two Hour Glucose Reading:_____

Mid Morning Snack:_____

Lunch:

Time:_____ Total Carbs:_____

_____

_____

_____

Two Hour Glucose Reading:_____

Mid Afternoon Snack:_____

Dinner:

Time:_____Total Carbs:_____

_____

_____

_____

Two Hour Glucose Reading:_____

Evening Snack:_____

Date:_____

A.M. Glucose Reading:_____

Breakfast:

Time:_____ Total Carbs:_____

_____
_____
_____

Two Hour Glucose Reading:_____
Mid Morning Snack:_____

Lunch:

Time:_____ Total Carbs:_____

_____
_____
_____

Two Hour Glucose Reading:_____
Mid Afternoon Snack:_____

Dinner:

Time:_____Total Carbs:_____

_____
_____
_____

Two Hour Glucose Reading:_____
Evening Snack:_____

Date:_____

A.M. Glucose Reading:_____

Breakfast:

Time:_____ Total Carbs:_____

_____
_____
_____

Two Hour Glucose Reading:_____
Mid Morning Snack:_____

Lunch:

Time:_____ Total Carbs:_____

_____
_____
_____

Two Hour Glucose Reading:_____
Mid Afternoon Snack:_____

Dinner:

Time:_____ Total Carbs:_____

_____
_____
_____

Two Hour Glucose Reading:_____
Evening Snack:_____

Date:_____

A.M. Glucose Reading:_____

Breakfast:

Time:_____    Total Carbs:_____
_____
_____
_____

Two Hour Glucose Reading:_____
Mid Morning Snack:_____

Lunch:

Time:_____    Total Carbs:_____
_____
_____
_____

Two Hour Glucose Reading:_____
Mid Afternoon Snack:_____

Dinner:

Time:_____Total Carbs:_____
_____
_____
_____

Two Hour Glucose Reading:_____
Evening Snack:_____

Date:_____

A.M. Glucose Reading:_____

---

Breakfast:

Time:_____ Total Carbs:_____

_____
_____
_____

Two Hour Glucose Reading:_____
Mid Morning Snack:_____

---

Lunch:

Time:_____ Total Carbs:_____

_____
_____
_____

Two Hour Glucose Reading:_____
Mid Afternoon Snack:_____

---

Dinner:

Time:_____Total Carbs:_____

_____
_____
_____

Two Hour Glucose Reading:_____
Evening Snack:_____

Date:_____

A.M. Glucose Reading:_____

---

Breakfast:

Time:_____  Total Carbs:_____

_____
_____
_____

Two Hour Glucose Reading:_____
Mid Morning Snack:_____

---

Lunch:

Time:_____  Total Carbs:_____

_____
_____
_____

Two Hour Glucose Reading:_____
Mid Afternoon Snack:_____

---

Dinner:

Time:_____Total Carbs:_____

_____
_____
_____

Two Hour Glucose Reading:_____
Evening Snack:_____

Date:_____

A.M. Glucose Reading:_____

---

Breakfast:

Time:_____   Total Carbs:_____

_____

_____

_____

Two Hour Glucose Reading:_____

Mid Morning Snack:_____

---

Lunch:

Time:_____   Total Carbs:_____

_____

_____

_____

Two Hour Glucose Reading:_____
Mid Afternoon Snack:_____

---

Dinner:

Time:_____Total Carbs:_____

_____

_____

_____

Two Hour Glucose Reading:_____
Evening Snack:_____

Date:_____

A.M. Glucose Reading:_____

Breakfast:

Time:_____ Total Carbs:_____

_____
_____
_____

Two Hour Glucose Reading:_____
Mid Morning Snack:_____

Lunch:

Time:_____ Total Carbs:_____

_____
_____
_____

Two Hour Glucose Reading:_____
Mid Afternoon Snack:_____

Dinner:

Time:_____Total Carbs:_____

_____
_____
_____

Two Hour Glucose Reading:_____
Evening Snack:_____

Date:_____

A.M. Glucose Reading:_____

Breakfast:

Time:_____ Total Carbs:_____
_____
_____
_____

Two Hour Glucose Reading:_____
Mid Morning Snack:_____

Lunch:

Time:_____ Total Carbs:_____
_____
_____
_____

Two Hour Glucose Reading:_____
Mid Afternoon Snack:_____

Dinner:

Time:_____Total Carbs:_____
_____
_____
_____

Two Hour Glucose Reading:_____
Evening Snack:_____

Date:_____

A.M. Glucose Reading:_____

Breakfast:

Time:_____ Total Carbs:_____
_____
_____
_____
Two Hour Glucose Reading:_____
Mid Morning Snack:_____

Lunch:

Time:_____ Total Carbs:_____
_____
_____
_____
Two Hour Glucose Reading:_____
Mid Afternoon Snack:_____

Dinner:

Time:_____Total Carbs:_____
_____
_____
_____
Two Hour Glucose Reading:_____
Evening Snack:_____

Date:_____

A.M. Glucose Reading:_____

Breakfast:

Time:_____ Total Carbs:_____

_____
_____
_____

Two Hour Glucose Reading:_____

Mid Morning Snack:_____

Lunch:

Time:_____ Total Carbs:_____

_____
_____
_____

Two Hour Glucose Reading:_____

Mid Afternoon Snack:_____

Dinner:

Time:_____Total Carbs:_____

_____
_____
_____

Two Hour Glucose Reading:_____

Evening Snack:_____

Date:_____

A.M. Glucose Reading:_____

---

Breakfast:

Time:_____    Total Carbs:_____

_____

_____

_____

Two Hour Glucose Reading:_____

Mid Morning Snack:_____

---

Lunch:

Time:_____    Total Carbs:_____

_____

_____

_____

Two Hour Glucose Reading:_____

Mid Afternoon Snack:_____

---

Dinner:

Time:_____Total Carbs:_____

_____

_____

_____

Two Hour Glucose Reading:_____

Evening Snack:_____

Date:_____

A.M. Glucose Reading:_____

Breakfast:

Time:_____ Total Carbs:_____

_____
_____
_____

Two Hour Glucose Reading:_____
Mid Morning Snack:_____

Lunch:

Time:_____ Total Carbs:_____

_____
_____
_____

Two Hour Glucose Reading:_____
Mid Afternoon Snack:_____

Dinner:

Time:_____Total Carbs:_____

_____
_____
_____

Two Hour Glucose Reading:_____
Evening Snack:_____

Date:_____

A.M. Glucose Reading:_____

Breakfast:

Time:_____ Total Carbs:_____
_____
_____
_____

Two Hour Glucose Reading:_____
Mid Morning Snack:_____

Lunch:

Time:_____ Total Carbs:_____
_____
_____
_____

Two Hour Glucose Reading:_____
Mid Afternoon Snack:_____

Dinner:

Time:_____Total Carbs:_____
_____
_____
_____

Two Hour Glucose Reading:_____
Evening Snack:_____

Date:_____

A.M. Glucose Reading:_____

Breakfast:

Time:_____ Total Carbs:_____

_____
_____
_____

Two Hour Glucose Reading:_____
Mid Morning Snack:_____

Lunch:

Time:_____ Total Carbs:_____

_____
_____
_____

Two Hour Glucose Reading:_____
Mid Afternoon Snack:_____

Dinner:

Time:_____Total Carbs:_____

_____
_____
_____

Two Hour Glucose Reading:_____
Evening Snack:_____

Date:_____

A.M. Glucose Reading:_____

Breakfast:

Time:_____ Total Carbs:_____

_____
_____
_____

Two Hour Glucose Reading:_____
Mid Morning Snack:_____

Lunch:

Time:_____ Total Carbs:_____

_____
_____
_____

Two Hour Glucose Reading:_____
Mid Afternoon Snack:_____

Dinner:

Time:_____Total Carbs:_____

_____
_____
_____

Two Hour Glucose Reading:_____
Evening Snack:_____

Date:_____

A.M. Glucose Reading:_____

Breakfast:

Time:_____ Total Carbs:_____
_____
_____
_____

Two Hour Glucose Reading:_____
Mid Morning Snack:_____

Lunch:

Time:_____ Total Carbs:_____
_____
_____
_____

Two Hour Glucose Reading:_____
Mid Afternoon Snack:_____

Dinner:

Time:_____Total Carbs:_____
_____
_____
_____

Two Hour Glucose Reading:_____
Evening Snack:_____

Date:_____

A.M. Glucose Reading:_____

Breakfast:

Time:_____ Total Carbs:_____

_____

_____

_____

Two Hour Glucose Reading:_____

Mid Morning Snack:_____

Lunch:

Time:_____ Total Carbs:_____

_____

_____

_____

Two Hour Glucose Reading:_____

Mid Afternoon Snack:_____

Dinner:

Time:_____Total Carbs:_____

_____

_____

_____

Two Hour Glucose Reading:_____

Evening Snack:_____

Date:_____

A.M. Glucose Reading:_____

---

Breakfast:

Time:_____ Total Carbs:_____

_____
_____
_____

Two Hour Glucose Reading:_____
Mid Morning Snack:_____

---

Lunch:

Time:_____ Total Carbs:_____

_____
_____
_____

Two Hour Glucose Reading:_____
Mid Afternoon Snack:_____

---

Dinner:

Time:_____Total Carbs:_____

_____
_____
_____

Two Hour Glucose Reading:_____
Evening Snack:_____

Date:_____

A.M. Glucose Reading:_____

---

Breakfast:

Time:_____ Total Carbs:_____

_____

_____

_____

Two Hour Glucose Reading:_____

Mid Morning Snack:_____

---

Lunch:

Time:_____ Total Carbs:_____

_____

_____

_____

Two Hour Glucose Reading:_____

Mid Afternoon Snack:_____

---

Dinner:

Time:_____Total Carbs:_____

_____

_____

_____

Two Hour Glucose Reading:_____

Evening Snack:_____

Date:_____

A.M. Glucose Reading:_____

Breakfast:

Time:_____ Total Carbs:_____

_____
_____
_____

Two Hour Glucose Reading:_____

Mid Morning Snack:_____

Lunch:

Time:_____ Total Carbs:_____

_____
_____
_____

Two Hour Glucose Reading:_____
Mid Afternoon Snack:_____

Dinner:

Time:_____Total Carbs:_____

_____
_____
_____

Two Hour Glucose Reading:_____
Evening Snack:_____

Date:_____

A.M. Glucose Reading:_____

Breakfast:

Time:_____ Total Carbs:_____

_____
_____
_____

Two Hour Glucose Reading:_____
Mid Morning Snack:_____

Lunch:

Time:_____ Total Carbs:_____

_____
_____
_____

Two Hour Glucose Reading:_____
Mid Afternoon Snack:_____

Dinner:

Time:_____Total Carbs:_____

_____
_____
_____

Two Hour Glucose Reading:_____
Evening Snack:_____

Date:_____

A.M. Glucose Reading:_____

Breakfast:

Time:_____ Total Carbs:_____

_____
_____
_____

Two Hour Glucose Reading:_____
Mid Morning Snack:_____

Lunch:

Time:_____ Total Carbs:_____

_____
_____
_____

Two Hour Glucose Reading:_____
Mid Afternoon Snack:_____

Dinner:

Time:_____Total Carbs:_____

_____
_____
_____

Two Hour Glucose Reading:_____
Evening Snack:_____

Date:_____

A.M. Glucose Reading:_____

Breakfast:

Time:_____ Total Carbs:_____

_____

_____

_____

Two Hour Glucose Reading:_____

Mid Morning Snack:_____

Lunch:

Time:_____ Total Carbs:_____

_____

_____

_____

Two Hour Glucose Reading:_____

Mid Afternoon Snack:_____

Dinner:

Time:_____Total Carbs:_____

_____

_____

_____

Two Hour Glucose Reading:_____

Evening Snack:_____

Date:_____

A.M. Glucose Reading:_____

Breakfast:

Time:_____  Total Carbs:_____

_____
_____
_____

Two Hour Glucose Reading:_____
Mid Morning Snack:_____

Lunch:

Time:_____  Total Carbs:_____

_____
_____
_____

Two Hour Glucose Reading:_____
Mid Afternoon Snack:_____

Dinner:

Time:_____Total Carbs:_____

_____
_____
_____

Two Hour Glucose Reading:_____
Evening Snack:_____

Date:_____

A.M. Glucose Reading:_____

---

**Breakfast:**

Time:_____ Total Carbs:_____

_____

_____

_____

Two Hour Glucose Reading:_____

Mid Morning Snack:_____

---

**Lunch:**

Time:_____ Total Carbs:_____

_____

_____

_____

Two Hour Glucose Reading:_____

Mid Afternoon Snack:_____

---

**Dinner:**

Time:_____Total Carbs:_____

_____

_____

_____

Two Hour Glucose Reading:_____

Evening Snack:_____

Date:_____

A.M. Glucose Reading:_____

---

Breakfast:

Time:_____  Total Carbs:_____

_____
_____
_____

Two Hour Glucose Reading:_____
Mid Morning Snack:_____

---

Lunch:

Time:_____  Total Carbs:_____

_____
_____
_____

Two Hour Glucose Reading:_____
Mid Afternoon Snack:_____

---

Dinner:

Time:_____Total Carbs:_____

_____
_____
_____

Two Hour Glucose Reading:_____
Evening Snack:_____

Date:_____

A.M. Glucose Reading:_____

---

Breakfast:

Time:_____ Total Carbs:_____

_____
_____
_____

Two Hour Glucose Reading:_____
Mid Morning Snack:_____

---

Lunch:

Time:_____ Total Carbs:_____

_____
_____
_____

Two Hour Glucose Reading:_____
Mid Afternoon Snack:_____

---

Dinner:

Time:_____Total Carbs:_____

_____
_____
_____

Two Hour Glucose Reading:_____
Evening Snack:_____

Date:_____

A.M. Glucose Reading:_____

---

Breakfast:

Time:_____ Total Carbs:_____

_____
_____
_____

Two Hour Glucose Reading:_____

Mid Morning Snack:_____

---

Lunch:

Time:_____ Total Carbs:_____

_____
_____
_____

Two Hour Glucose Reading:_____

Mid Afternoon Snack:_____

---

Dinner:

Time:_____Total Carbs:_____

_____
_____
_____

Two Hour Glucose Reading:_____

Evening Snack:_____

Date:_____

A.M. Glucose Reading:_____

---

Breakfast:

Time:_____    Total Carbs:_____
_____
_____
_____

Two Hour Glucose Reading:_____
Mid Morning Snack:_____

---

Lunch:

Time:_____    Total Carbs:_____
_____
_____
_____

Two Hour Glucose Reading:_____
Mid Afternoon Snack:_____

---

Dinner:

Time:_____Total Carbs:_____
_____
_____
_____

Two Hour Glucose Reading:_____
Evening Snack:_____

Date:_____

A.M. Glucose Reading:_____

Breakfast:

Time:_____ Total Carbs:_____

_____
_____
_____

Two Hour Glucose Reading:_____
Mid Morning Snack:_____

Lunch:

Time:_____ Total Carbs:_____

_____
_____
_____

Two Hour Glucose Reading:_____
Mid Afternoon Snack:_____

Dinner:

Time:_____Total Carbs:_____

_____
_____
_____

Two Hour Glucose Reading:_____
Evening Snack:_____